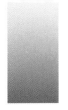

TABLE OF CONTENTS

2

APPENDIX 3

APPENDIX 4

PREFACE

It gives me great pleasure to write the Preface for this the 7th Annual Report of the Confidential Enquiry into Stillbirths & Deaths in Infancy (CESDI).

Since taking responsibility for the organisation and running of the Enquiry, the Maternal & Child Health Research Consortium (MCHRC), established by the Royal College of Midwives, Royal College of Obstetricians & Gynaecologists, Royal College of Paediatrics & Child Health and the Royal College of Pathologists, have further developed the methodologies and scope of the Enquiry. Confidential enquiries could be criticised for looking only at uncommon and fatal outcomes out of context to the totality of service provision. CESDI has addressed this through the introduction of case-control studies and, this year, the collection of denominator data. The rolling programme changes regularly within a two year period. Each topic requires different data collection mechanisms and more specifically a unique structured enquiry form for the panels to utilise. Inevitably these take time to develop and pilot, and training is required at regional level to ensure appropriate use and speedy data collection.

Having the four Royal Colleges involved in the Consortium has ensured a sense of ownership of the enquiry findings and means that the recommendations from the various aspects of work undertaken can be quickly taken forward by the Colleges. The recommendations are being incorporated into their guidelines and working party structures; this ensures widespread dissemination, and aids uptake into clinical practice with resultant change and improved standards of care.

To run such a complex, unique and effective Enquiry requires appropriate resourcing and a dedicated team of staff. These include individuals directing policy, a central Secretariat, the all-important Regional Co-ordinators, district-based data collectors and the enquiry panel members. Each individual is an integral link in ensuring a successful outcome to our enquiry process.

CESDI is nearing the end of its five year contract with the Department of Health and is looking forward to developing its work within NICE. CESDI can then continue to contribute effectively to providing explanations for many stillbirths, neonatal deaths and deaths in the first year of life. It will seek to provide guidance to professionals to enable them to make further improvements to what for the most part are already high standards of care.

I hope you will find the issues highlighted in this 7th Report interesting, relevant and applicable within your sphere of practice.

PROFESSOR ROBERT W SHAW
Chairman - Maternal & Child Health Research Consortium (MCHRC)
President - Royal College of Obstetricians & Gynaecologists

MEMBERS OF THE CESDI ORGANISATION

MEMBERS OF THE MATERNAL & CHILD HEALTH RESEARCH CONSORTIUM (MCHRC) EXECUTIVE STEERING GROUP

Professor Robert Shaw (Chair)
Royal College of Obstetricians & Gynaecologists

Ms Polly Ferguson
Royal College of Midwives

Dr Steve Gould
Royal College of Pathologists

Dr Patricia Hamilton
Royal College of Paediatrics & Child Health

Professor Martin Whittle
Royal College of Obstetricians & Gynaecologists

MEMBERS OF THE INTERIM ADVISORY GROUP

Professor Andrew Wilkinson (Chair), Professor of Paediatrics, University of Oxford

Mrs Vicky Bailey
Senior Midwife
Nottingham Health Authority

Miss Sue Burr, OBE
Adviser on Paediatric Nursing
Royal College of Nursing

Dr Patrick Cartlidge
Consultant Neonatal Paediatrician
University of Wales College of Medicine

Dr Jean Chapple
Consultant Perinatal Epidemiologist
Kensington, Chelsea and Westminster
Health Authority

Mr Andrew Dillon
Chief Executive, National Institute for
Clinical Excellence

Dr James Dornan
Consultant Obstetrician
Royal Maternity Hospital, Belfast

Professor Keith Greene
Consultant Obstetrician and Gynaecologist
Derriford Hospital, Plymouth

Ms Patricia Hanson
CESDI Regional Co-ordinator
South East Thames

Mrs Eileen Hutton, OBE
Parental Voice

Dr Jean Keeling
Consultant Paediatric Pathologist
Royal Hospital for Sick Children,
Edinburgh

Dr Mark Lambert
Consultant in Public Health Medicine
Gateshead and South Tyneside Health
Authority

Mrs Linda Lamont
Parental Voice

Dr Roddy Macfaul
Medical Advisor, Paediatric and
Children's Health Services,
Department of Health

Mrs Stephanie Meakin
Practice Development Co-ordinator
Royal College of Midwives

Professor Robert Shaw
Chair - Maternal and Child Health
Research Consortium

Professor Martin Whittle
Consultant Obstetrician
Birmingham Women's Hospital

Dr Gavin Young
General Practitioner
Temple Sowerby, Cumbria

THE CESDI SECRETARIAT

Director	**Dr Mary Macintosh**
Project Manager	**Ms Helen Caddy**
Midwife	**Mrs Niki Jakeman**
Midwife (until February 2000)	**Mrs Cathy Winter**
Midwife (from January 2000)	**Mrs Sian Warriner**
IT Specialist	**Mr Charles Lee**
Data Analyst	**Ms Joy Lawrence**
Data Analyst	**Mr Steven Bailey**
Secretary	**Mrs Mary Humphreys**

THE CESDI REGIONAL CO-ORDINATORS

Northern	**Ms Marjorie Renwick**
Yorkshire	**Ms Lesley Anson**
Trent	**Ms Sue Wood**
Anglia	**Ms Jane Baker (until January 2000) Ms Carol Hay**
North West Thames	**Ms Stephanie Roberts**
North East Thames	**Ms Dawn Saunders (until February 2000) Ms Sarah Das**
South East Thames	**Ms Patricia Hanson**
South Thames West	**Ms Sharon Hackett (until May 2000) Ms Julia Chachere**
Wessex and The Channel Islands	**Ms Melanie Gompels**
Oxford	**Ms Irene Boller**
South Western	**Ms Rosie Thompson**
West Midlands	**Ms Donna Drinkall**

sey	**Ms Grace Edwards**
North Western	**Dr Jean Sands**
Wales	**Ms Jane Stewart**
Northern Ireland	**Dr Maureen Scott** **Ms Terry Falconer**

1

INTRODUCTION

1.1 **HISTORY**

The Confidential Enquiry into Stillbirths and Deaths in Infancy (CESDI) was established in 1992 to improve understanding of how the risks of death in late fetal life up to infancy might be reduced. CESDI seeks to identify and highlight risks which can be attributed to suboptimal clinical care.

In 1991 the Department of Health directed that the fourteen 'Regions' of England should undertake Perinatal Mortality Surveys. CESDI was subsequently organised on this regional basis with separate arrangements for Wales and Northern Ireland. The CESDI network has remained despite organisational changes in the NHS during 1994-95 and 1998-99.

Initially, CESDI was funded directly by the Department of Health and supervised by a National Advisory Body (NAB), under the chairmanship of Lady Littler. In April 1996 responsibility for the management of CESDI was assumed by the Maternal and Child Health Research Consortium (MCHRC). This group was established by the Royal College of Obstetricians & Gynaecologists, Royal College of Paediatrics & Child Health, Royal College of Pathology and the Royal College of Midwives, to oversee the running of the Enquiry. As from April 1st 1999 CESDI is one of the four National Enquiries under the umbrella of the National Institute for Clinical Excellence (NICE). NICE has commissioned a review of the role of the Confidential Enquiries and in particular their impact on health care. This review is timely as there is a need to optimise the ways that enquiry processes lead to improved practice. It is anticipated that NICE will appoint an Advisory Body to fulfil the role of the NAB. Meanwhile the Interim Advisory Group has been established until these arrangements are implemented.

In England, Wales and Northern Ireland there are some 10,000 deaths annually occurring between 20 weeks gestation and 1 year of life. Data on each of these deaths is collected locally, using a rapid reporting notification system (RRF) and passed to the Regional Co-ordinator. These are collated at the CESDI Secretariat. A sub-set are enquired into by multidisciplinary panels within regions.

The CESDI Secretariat is responsible for the design, piloting and implementation of the work programmes; the collation, analysis and reporting of the findings to provide a comprehensive national overview, and the preparation and dissemination of the CESDI Annual Report.

1.2 **THE WORK OF CESDI**

CESDI is tasked to provide an overview of the numbers and causes of stillbirth and infant deaths, together with a detailed enquiry into specific sub-sets. A variety of approaches have been used: case control studies where risk factors need to be assessed; focus group work to provide greater detail and overview of rare events. CESDI has also undertaken several audits evaluating whether its recommendations are implemented. Table 1.1 summarises the programme to date. In addition, CESDI in collaboration with various agencies, including the Royal Colleges, has produced two information leaflets; A Guide to the Postmortem Examination - Brief Notes for Parents (1998) and The Fetal and Infant Postmortem - Brief Notes for the Professional (1999), which have been widely distributed, and are available on the CESDI website, www.cesdi.org.uk.

Table 1.1 The work programmes of CESDI

Enquiry Topic	Year of study	Findings Reported
Intrapartum related deaths >2.5 kg	1993	2nd Annual Report
Intrapartum related deaths > 1.5 kg	1994-1995	4th Annual Report
'Explained' Sudden Unexpected Deaths in Infancy	1993-1996	5th Annual Report
.1 in 10 sample of all deaths >1kg	1996-1997	6th Annual Report
All deaths 4 kg and over	1997	6th Annual Report
Case Control Studies		
Sudden Unexpected Deaths in Infancy	1993-1994	3rd Annual Report
Sudden Unexpected Deaths in Infancy	1993-1996	The CESDI SUDI studies[1]
Antepartum Term Stillbirths	1995	5th Annual Report
Project 27-28	1998-2000	To be reported
Focus Groups		
Shoulder dystocia	1994-1995	5th Annual Report
Ruptured uterus	1994-1995	5th Annual Report
Planned home delivery	1994-1995	5th Annual Report
Anaesthetic complications and delays	1994-1995	7th Annual Report
Breech presentation at onset of labour	1994-1995	7th Annual Report
Audits		
Postmortem reporting	1993	2nd Annual Report
Postmortem reporting	1994-1995	6th Annual Report
CTG education	1999	7th Annual Report

1.3   **THE METHODOLOGY**

Essential components of the process include:

i   A rapid and validated notification system.

ii   External and independent multidisciplinary enquiry

iii   Standardisation of the enquiry process

The initial enquiries involved only deaths and limited the scope of the interpretation of the findings in a wider context. In response to this, 'denominators' and controls were introduced into the current programme on the care of premature babies (Project 27/28) in 1998.

1.4   **ENQUIRY PROCESS**
        The enquiry comprises a review of the complete set of anonymised
        medical records by a multidisciplinary panel not involved with the
        case or hospital. Each panel consists of experts from a number of
        disciplines including obstetrics, paediatrics, midwifery, specialist
        perinatal/paediatric pathology and general practice. Other parties
        with appropriate expertise may also be involved. Panel members are
        sent anonymised case-notes prior to the meeting. At the meeting itself
        the panel produce a summary of the case and complete a standard
        CESDI form outlining any areas of suboptimal care.

        The information is given with the understanding that there will be no
        feedback to the units or individuals concerned with the case but that
        the findings will be published in a Report.

        Over time the panel enquiry process has been modified to improve its
        consistency of appraisal. This has included introduction of a
        structured enquiry form and guidance on the standards of care being
        assessed.

        The multidisciplinary and independent nature of the panel provides
        an optimum setting for identifying errors of care and focuses on
        systems rather than individuals.

1.5   **CURRENT ENQUIRY PROGRAMME - PROJECT 27/28**
        Prematurity is the major cause of neonatal deaths, especially in babies
        weighing less than 1.5kg, who account for 1-2% of births, but
        approximately half of all neonatal deaths. This group is also a major
        contributor to long term neurological disability. Despite growing
        professional and public interest in the care given to babies born before
        32 weeks' gestation there is no national information. This is because
        gestational age at birth is not routinely collected on all live births in
        England, Wales and Northern Ireland.

        CESDI is currently identifying all babies born in the 27 to 28 weeks'
        gestational range to provide denominator data for survival figures.
        Confidential enquiries are being held on all neonatal deaths and an
        equivalent number of the randomly selected survivors in this
        gestational range. These findings will identify areas of suboptimal care
        up to the first seven days of life associated with death of these babies.

        The aims and objectives and a detailed description of Project 27/28 are
        outlined in the 6th Annual Report.

1.5.1   **Project 27/28 - The first year**
        In the first year CESDI received notification of 3822 babies via logs
        placed on 339 labour wards and neonatal units in England, Wales and
        Northern Ireland. These relate to liveborn babies born between 1st
        September 1998 and 31st August 1999 with a clinical gestation of 26^{+0} to
        29^{+6} weeks. Of these 1834 were in the 27^{+0} to 28^{+6} weeks' gestational
        range according to the dating algorithm, with 1386 (76%) singleton
        and 448 (24%) multiple babies. Survival rates at day 28 for this cohort
        are given in Table 1.2.

Transfers out of the first neonatal unit occurred in 29% (526/1834) of the babies at gestational age 27^{+0} to 28^{+6} weeks within 28 days, and in 9% (172/1834) within the first 48 hours.

Table 1.2. Notifications and survival rates of liveborn babies at 27^{+0} to 28^{+6} weeks gestation born between 01/09/98 to 31/08/99 in England, Wales and Northern Ireland.

	Notifications (%)	Alive at day 28	Survival rate at day 28 (%)
Singletons	1386 (76%)	1213	87.5%
Multiples	448 (24%)	388	86.6%
Overall	1834 (100%)	1601	87.3%

CESDI has produced a poster and leaflet giving information on data collected in the first year of the Project. This is available on the CESDI website www.cesdi.org.uk

1.5.2 Project 27/28 - The second year

During the design of the Project, a survival rate of 80% for babies at 27/28 weeks gestation had been anticipated and an estimated 263 neonatal deaths per year. It was initially planned, due to workload restrictions, to limit the enquiries to babies dying within the first 7 days (early neonatal deaths). During data collection, it became apparent that the survival rate was higher than expected (87.3 %) and so late neonatal deaths for both years have been included for enquiry.

For the first year cohort, enquiries were conducted within the region of birth but for the second year's cohort, enquiries will be pooled and allocated out of region. This is to overcome the difficulties in providing neonatologists not involved with the case for the panel assessment, and to increase the variety of cases reviewed locally.

1.6 FUTURE WORK PROGRAMME

Perinatal death in multiple pregnancies is 4 to 5 times that of singletons. There are over 9000 multiple maternities in England, Wales and Northern Ireland each year, accounting for about 1.5% of deliveries but they contribute disproportionately (10% of notifications to CESDI) to stillbirths, infant deaths and very low birth weights. The incidence of twinning in the UK has increased from 9.9/1000 maternities (5909 twin maternities) in 1975 to 14.5/1000 (8899 twin maternities) in 1997[2, 3]. There is no consensus regarding optimum management for these pregnancies and deliveries. There have been several developments in the last ten years, in particular risk assessment by ultrasound determination of chorionicity in early pregnancy. This is widely held to help identify pregnancies at particular risk of complications. However, the actual benefit of early diagnosis remains unknown. Policies of antenatal surveillance for twin pregnancies vary and the extent to which this contributes to fetal or neonatal loss is unknown. For these reasons the Interim Advisory Group has chosen Multiple Pregnancies as the topic for the next National Enquiry programme.

Preliminary work is also underway reviewing the optimum methods of enquiring into infant deaths that occur in hospital following an admission. Each year there are over four hundred such deaths. In this group it is particularly important to assess the care pathway from home into the hospital.

1.7 **CONTENTS OF THIS REPORT**

1.7.1 **Infant and Perinatal Mortality - 1998**
CESDI undertakes a national on-going survey of perinatal and infant deaths (between 20 weeks' gestation and 1 year). The information collected is clinical and differs from that collected at the time of registration by the Office for National Statistics. Chapter 2 summarises 1998 notifications, and highlights trends from 1993.

1.7.2 **Focus Group - Breech presentation at onset of labour**
The management of breech presentation is a contentious issue. Despite a lack of supportive data there is an increasing use of Caesarean section as the routine mode of delivery in the UK. This has resulted in fewer training opportunities and current experience in the management of vaginal breech deliveries. Breech presentation is known to be associated with a higher perinatal mortality and morbidity due to prematurity, congenital malformations and birth asphyxia or trauma. For these reasons death associated with vaginal breech at onset of labour was chosen to be the subject of a Focus Group report (Chapter 3) providing an overview of these events.

1.7.3 **Focus Group - Obstetric anaesthesia - delays and complications**
The death of a baby as a result of an event in labour is a rare (approximately 1 in 1500 deliveries) and traumatic event. In 1994 and 1995 all such cases (873) underwent a panel enquiry. Although the anaesthetic care rarely contributed directly to these deaths, there were several instances associated with significant difficulties in the provision of the anaesthetic. These included technical problems in administration, delays with personnel and delays in the provision of anaesthesia once the anaesthetist was available. These events are the subject of a Focus Group report in Chapter 4.

1.7.4 **Cardiotocograph education survey**
The review of the intrapartum related deaths in 1994-1995 concluded that half of the deaths were likely to have been avoided with alternative management (4th Annual Report). The most frequent criticism related to failures in the use and interpretation of cardiotocograph (CTG) tracings. CESDI recommended that every hospital offering intrapartum care should have in place a training programme in the use of CTGs for all professionals (4th Annual Report, 1997). This year CESDI undertook a survey to determine if these recommendations were being followed. The results are reported in Chapter 5.

1.7.5 Sudden unexpected deaths in infancy - pathology

In 1993 to 1996 CESDI undertook the largest study to date on sudden unexpected deaths in infancy. A full account and the overall findings have been published separately[1]. One of the main conclusions is that a thorough postmortem is essential in these circumstances. A summary of the main pathology findings of the 450 postmortems is given in Chapter 6. This work resulted in a recommended postmortem protocol for such cases.

1.7.6 Communication

Previous CESDI Reports have drawn attention to the significant contribution to suboptimal care made by deficiencies in communications. Communication failures were cited in some 17% of the comments analysed for the three years of the enquiries into intrapartum related deaths (2nd and 4th Annual Reports). CESDI commissioned a review of published evidence of the contribution of these failures to perinatal losses. A summary of this review is given in Chapter 7.

1.7.7 Changing local practice

The findings of CESDI need to be acted on as well as understood. The last two Reports (5th and 6th) included a review of how at a National level the Royal Colleges and other statutory bodies responsible for training and accreditation are responding to the recommendations. This year we have undertaken a similar exercise at Regional level and the results are reported in Chapter 8.

1.8 VIEWS OF THE INTERIM ADVISORY GROUP

The Interim Advisory Group have been consulted about this Report and are in agreement with contents.

1.9 FEEDBACK FROM READERS

CESDI welcomes feedback from readers and a questionnaire is enclosed with the Report seeking views. In addition, readers are asked to comment on any aspect of the Report, or the work of CESDI via the CESDI Website on www.cesdi.org.uk

REFERENCES

1.   Fleming P, Blair P, Bacon C, Berry J. Sudden Unexpected Deaths In Infancy; The CESDI SUDI Studies 1993-1996. London: The Stationery Office, 2000.

2.   Dunn A, Macfarlane A. Recent trends in the incidence of multiple births and associated mortality in England and Wales. Archives of disease in Childhood, 1996;75: 10-19

3.   ONS. Birth statistics 1997 - England and Wales. Series FM1 no.26 London: The Stationery Office, 1998.

ACKNOWLEDGEMENTS

Members of the Consortium Executive Steering Group, the Secretariat, the National Advisory Body, the Interim Advisory Group and the various working groups are listed in the Report. While it has been the prime responsibility of the Secretariat and the Executive Steering Group to produce the Report, they gratefully acknowledge the invaluable input made by the Interim Advisory Group to the Report as a whole, as well as the other contributors named in the footnotes to individual chapters.

2

INFANT AND PERINATAL MORTALITY - 1998

2.1   INTRODUCTION

The Rapid Report Form (RRF) is the CESDI notification system first used in 1993. Its purposes are:

- To obtain a dataset for each death within the CESDI range between 20 weeks gestation and one year of life.
- To provide information as soon as possible after the death in order to support the enquiry process.

The RRF data collection form for 1998 is reproduced in Appendix 2.

A national collection of mortality statistics is also conducted by the Office for National Statistics (ONS) based on registered deaths of babies born from 24 weeks onwards. This comprises socio-demographic and occupational details and is collected from the Registrar of Births and Deaths. As registration of death is statutory, the ONS figures form the gold standard for comparison with the RRF returns. The content of RRF data is predominantly clinical.

2.2   NOTIFICATIONS TO CESDI

2.2.1   Ascertainment and quality of CESDI notifications

Ascertainment of CESDI notifications has improved consistently since 1993 and has levelled at around 99% from 1996 onwards. Identification of postneonatal deaths has been the most difficult for CESDI and this has continued to improve from 86% in 1993, to 96% in 1998.

The quality of the data items on the RRF is assessed by the response rate to 29 questions considered to be essential. In general completion of these questions was high, for example - case definition (100%), date delivered (99.8%), date of death (99.9%), sex (98.2%) Wigglesworth classification (99.1%). The least well answered question was the first date of the last menstrual period (87.5%).

2.2.2   Stillbirth and neonatal death rates

Table 2.1 shows the number of deaths reported to CESDI by RRF between 1993 and 1998. The stillbirth rate shows a steady decrease since 1995 and the neonatal rate since 1996.

Table 2.1: Rapid Report Form returns 1993 - 1998

| | England, Wales and Northern Ireland | | | | | | | | | | | |
| | 1993 | | 1994 | | 1995 | | 1996 | | 1997 | | 1998 | |
	Numbers	Rate	Numbers	Rate	Numbers	Rate	Numbers	Rate	Numbers	Rate	Numbers	Rate
Legal abortions	-		-		959	-	1102	-	1299	-	**1503**	-
Late fetal loss	1495	-	1573	-	1553	-	1659	-	1774	-	**1672**	-
(excl legal ab.) *legal abortions*									*1062*		*1204*	
*Stillbirths*¹	3726	5.3	3747	5.4	3698	5.5	3688	5.4	3440	5.1	**3347**	5.0
(excl legal ab.) *legal abortions*									*179*	*0.3*	*256*	*0.4*
*Perinatal deaths*¹	-	-	5897	8.5	5829	8.6	5898	8.7	5503	8.2	**5266**	7.9
(excl legal ab.) *legal abortions*									*237*	*0.4*	*299*	*0.5*
Neonatal deaths²	2755	4.0	2749	4.0	2714	4.0	2785	4.1	2648	4.0	**2493**	3.8
(excl legal ab.) *legal abortions*									*58*	*0.1*	*43*	*0.1*
Postneonatal deaths²	1242	1.8	1199	1.7	1156	1.7	1253	1.9	1257	1.9	**1210**	1.8
Total Reports - RRF	9218		9268		10080		10487		10418		**10225**	
Live births	696133		688545		671861		674071		666370		**659762**	

¹Rate per 1000 live births+stillbirths
²Rate per 1000 live births

Sources: Deaths: RRF 1998
Live Births: ONS Registrations 1998
N Ireland GRO 1998

Classification of legal abortions

Since 1995 CESDI has collected information on legal abortions after twenty weeks gestation. Up to 1996 the data did not distinguish between a legal abortion and a late fetal loss, stillbirth or early neonatal death. For example, if a late fetal loss was legally aborted, it could be reported as a late fetal loss or a legal abortion but not both. In 1997 the question on legal abortion was modified to enable it to be identified independently. Figure 2.1 shows the proportions of legal abortions for each case definition in 1998. The effects of these modifications on stillbirth, perinatal and neonatal death rates are shown in Table 2.1.

Figure 2.1: Legal abortions (1503) as a proportion of RRF returns (10225) - 1998

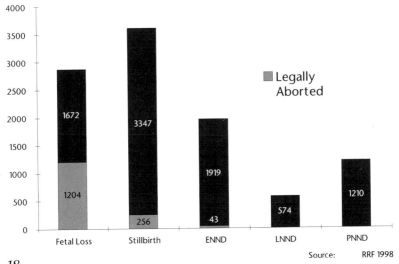

Source: RRF 1998

18

The numbers of livebirths, deaths and mortality rates for singleton and multiple births in England, Wales and Northern Ireland is shown in Table 2.2.

Table 2.2: Stillbirth and Neonatal deaths for singleton and multiple births 1993 - 1998

	England, Wales and Northern Ireland					
	1993	1994	1995	1996	1997	1998
Total live births	696133	688545	671861	674071	666370	659762
Singleton	678676	670734	653278	655834	647279	640781
Multiple	17457	17811	18583	18237	19091	18778
Stillbirths						
Singleton	3422	3390	3340	3329	3251	3230
Multiple	297	355	356	350	358	371
Unclassified	7	2	2	9	10	2
Neonatal deaths						
Singleton	2267	2259	2213	2258	2228	2071
Multiple	477	477	487	517	472	457
Unclassified	11	13	14	10	6	8
Stillbirth rate[1]						
Singleton	5.0	5.0	5.1	5.1	5.0	5.0
Multiple	16.7	19.5	18.8	18.8	18.4	19.4
Neonatal mortality rate[2]						
Singleton	3.3	3.4	3.4	3.4	3.4	3.2
Multiple	27.3	26.8	26.2	28.3	24.7	24.3

[1]Rate per 1000 live births+stillbirths
[2]Rate per 1000 live births

Sources: RRF 1998
ONS Registrations 1998
N Ireland GRO 1998

2.2.3 Cause of death

The cause of death according to the three classifications used by CESDI (the extended Wigglesworth; Obstetric Aberdeen; Fetal and Neonatal classification: Appendix 3) for stillbirths, neonatal and postneonatal deaths in 1998 is shown in Figures 2.2, 2.3, 2.4

For stillbirths according to the Wigglesworth classification (Figure 2.2), the largest proportion was unexplained antepartum fetal death (n=2521, 70.0%). The most common identifiable causes of death were congenital malformation (n=439, 12.2%) and intrapartum related events (n=330, 9.2%). The 2521 unexplained antepartum fetal deaths were further described using the Obstetric Aberdeen classification. This analysis indicated antepartum haemorrhage occurred in 395 cases.

For neonatal deaths according to the Wigglesworth classification (Figure 2.3), the main cause of death was immaturity (n=1231, 48.5%), followed by congenital malformation (n=582, 22.9%). The 1231 neonatal deaths caused by immaturity were further described using the Fetal and Neonatal classification, and 718 deaths of these were due to asphyxia before birth.

For postneonatal deaths (Figure 2.4), the three most common causes of death were congenital malformation (n=343, 28.3%), Sudden infant death (SIDs n=318, 26.3%), and infection (n=202, 16.7%).

Figure 2.2 Stillbirths in England, Wales and Northern Ireland by Wigglesworth classification - 1998

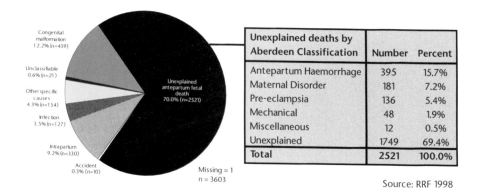

Unexplained deaths by Aberdeen Classification	Number	Percent
Antepartum Haemorrhage	395	15.7%
Maternal Disorder	181	7.2%
Pre-eclampsia	136	5.4%
Mechanical	48	1.9%
Miscellaneous	12	0.5%
Unexplained	1749	69.4%
Total	**2521**	**100.0%**

Source: RRF 1998

Figure 2.3 Neonatal deaths in England, Wales and Northern Ireland by Wigglesworth classification - 1998

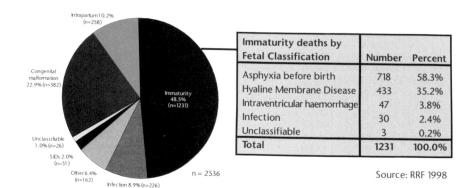

Immaturity deaths by Fetal Classification	Number	Percent
Asphyxia before birth	718	58.3%
Hyaline Membrane Disease	433	35.2%
Intraventricular haemorrhage	47	3.8%
Infection	30	2.4%
Unclassifiable	3	0.2%
Total	**1231**	**100.0%**

Source: RRF 1998

Figure 2.4 Postneonatal deaths in England, Wales and Northern Ireland by Wigglesworth classification - 1998

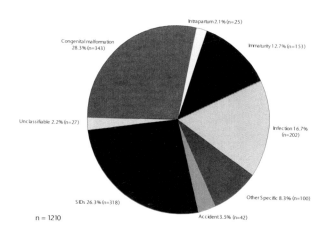

Source: RRF 1998

20

2.2.4 CESDI Mortality rates - Regional variation

Stillbirth, neonatal and postneonatal mortality rates by region of residence of mother in 1998 are shown in Figure 2.5. The source of the denominator data was the ONS (1998) and Northern Ireland GRO (1998). The ONS data pertaining to England were initially classified according to the eight NHS Executive Regional Office boundaries (1997) and converted to the 14 CESDI regions. Due to boundary changes, however, the conversion for some regions, notably South Western and Wessex and The Channel Islands are not exact. These crude mortality rates are **not** direct indicators of standards of care and should **not** be interpreted as such. There are other factors which influence outcomes.

The combined mortality rate (stillbirths, neonatal and postneonatal deaths per 1000 total births) was calculated for each region (Figure 2.5). This ranged from 9.5 to 12.4 deaths per 1000 total births and overall was 11.1 per 1000 total births. For comparison, figures have been included from the Scottish Stillbirth and Infant Report 1998.

Figure 2.5: Stillbirth[1], neonatal[2], postneonatal[2] and combined mortality rates by CESDI region of residence of mother - 1998

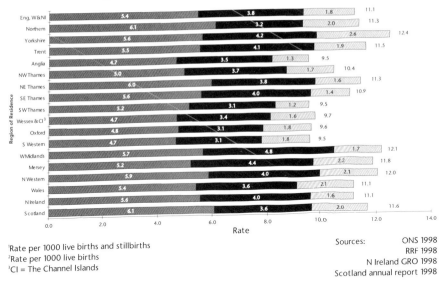

[1] Rate per 1000 live births and stillbirths
[2] Rate per 1000 live births
[3] CI = The Channel Islands

Sources: ONS 1998
RRF 1998
N Ireland GRO 1998
Scotland annual report 1998

2.2.5 Postmortem rates

The numbers and rates of postmortem examination for late fetal losses, stillbirths, neonatal and postneonatal deaths from the 1998 RRF returns are shown in Table 2.3. The overall postmortem rate for England, Wales and Northern Ireland was 55.1% and ranged from 44.7% to 67.2% within the CESDI regions. Stillbirths (61.5%) were the category most likely to have a postmortem and neonatal deaths the least likely (41.2%).

The rates for previous years are shown in Table 2.4.

Of the 5632 postmortems reported in 1998, 620 had been requested by a coroner.

The reasons for failure to perform a postmortem in 4269 cases were examined: offered but declined by parents or family (2534, 59.4%); not offered (1683, 39.4%); permission given but not performed (52, 1.2%). No information about postmortem (324, 3.2%).

Table 2.3: Numbers of, and percentages with postmortems of late fetal losses, stillbirths, neonatal and postneonatal deaths - 1998

REGION	Late fetal loss (incl terminations)		Stillbirths		Neonatal deaths		Postneonatal deaths		All deaths	
	Number	%PM	Number	%PM	Number	%PM	Number	%PM	Number	%PM
Eng, W & NI	2876	60.4	3603	61.5	2536	41.2	1210	52.3	10225	55.1
Northern	160	68.8	197	65.0	102	52.9	67	59.7	526	63.1
Yorkshire	170	61.2	229	52.4	178	29.2	112	48.2	689	47.9
Trent	171	59.1	319	60.2	232	43.1	106	57.5	828	54.8
Anglia	136	50.0	158	58.9	119	50.4	36	58.3	449	53.9
NW Thames	227	63.9	210	70.0	152	50.0	76	56.6	665	61.8
NE Thames	297	52.9	338	56.2	237	37.1	118	40.7	990	48.8
SE Thames	252	55.2	301	58.1	219	43.8	89	47.2	861	52.5
SW Thames	198	61.1	207	67.6	103	45.6	46	45.7	554	59.4
Wessex & CI[1]	131	69.5	165	69.1	113	54.9	56	73.2	465	66.2
Oxford	129	63.6	167	67.7	99	37.4	54	53.7	449	58.1
S Western	154	75.3	175	72.0	112	57.1	68	52.9	509	67.2
W Midlands	324	62.0	384	58.9	324	35.2	113	41.6	1145	51.4
Mersey	107	55.1	151	68.2	136	34.6	69	50.7	463	52.7
N Western	235	42.1	299	50.2	201	32.3	100	59.0	835	44.7
Wales	127	86.6	171	64.3	115	34.8	64	60.9	477	62.7
N Ireland	58	56.9	132	68.2	94	46.8	36	47.2	320	57.5

[1]CI = The Channel Islands

Source: RRF 1998

Table 2.4: Rates of postmortem performed - 1993 to 1998

National	Late fetal loss	Stillbirth	Neonatal deaths	Post neonatal deaths	All deaths
Year	%PM	%PM	%PM	%PM	%PM
1998	60.4	61.5	41.2	52.3	55.1
1997	57.5	61.6	40.7	56.2	54.4
1996	63.5	62.8	44.0	57.4	57.4
1995	57.5	64.1	46.0	57.5	56.6
1994	58.7	67.5	46.7	59.5	58.8
1993	54.2	66.7	47.6	60.3	58.1

Source: RRF 1998

1. **Total births and deaths:** Registered live births in England, Wales and Northern Ireland totalled 659762 in 1998. A total of 10225 deaths were notified to CESDI, comprising 1503 legal abortions, 2876 late fetal losses, 3603 stillbirths, 2536 neonatal deaths and 1210 postneonatal deaths.

2. **Stillbirths:** The stillbirth rate has steadily decreased since 1995. The rate was 5.0 per 1000 total births. This excludes legal abortions.

3. **Perinatal mortality rate:** 7.9 per 1000 total births. This excludes legal abortions.

4. **Neonatal death rate:** 3.8 per 1000 total births. This excludes legal abortions.

5. **Postneonatal mortality rate:** 1.8 per 1000 live births.

6. **Singleton births:** The stillbirth rate was 5.0 per 1000 singleton total births and the neonatal death rate was 3.2 per 1000 singleton live births.

7. **Multiple births:** The stillbirth rate was 19.4 per 1000 multiple total births and the neonatal death rate was 24.3 per 1000 multiple live births.

8. **CESDI Regional mortality rates:** The combined (stillbirth, neonatal and post-neonatal) mortality rate for England, Wales and Northern Ireland was 11.1 per 1000 total births and ranged from 9.5 to 12.4 within the regions.

9. **Postmortem examinations:** The overall postmortem rate for England, Wales and Northern Ireland was 55.1% (range: 44.7% - 67.2%). Within the various categories, the highest rate was 61.5% for stillbirths (range: 50.2% - 72.0%); the lowest rate 41.3% for neonatal deaths (range: 29.2% - 57.1%).

ACKNOWLEDGEMENTS

Authors:
Mr Steven Bailey, Data Analyst , CESDI Secretariat
Mr Charles Lee, IT Specialist, CESDI Secretariat

With thanks to :
Ms Nirupa Dattani (ONS) and Ms Terry Falconer (N Ireland) for providing denominator data.
Ms Nicola Cooper (ONS) for providing ascertainment checks.

3

FOCUS GROUP - BREECH PRESENTATION AT ONSET OF LABOUR

3.1 **BACKGROUND**

Breech presentation is known to be associated with a higher than normal perinatal mortality and morbidity due to prematurity, congenital malformations, birth asphyxia and trauma[1]. There is a commonly held belief that the latter, birth trauma, is responsible for a substantial part of the excess risk. Consequently, and despite a lack of supportive data, there is increasing use of Caesarean section as the routine mode of delivery in the UK. This has resulted in fewer training opportunities and thus less experience in the management of vaginal breech deliveries. Because of these issues death associated with breech presentation at the onset of labour was chosen as the subject of a focus group report.

3.2 **METHOD**

3.2.1 **Identification of cases**

CESDI has reported the findings of enquiries on all (873) normally formed babies weighing 1.5kg or over at birth who died as a result of an intrapartum event in 1994-1995[2]. Within this group there were 56 singleton babies that were breech presentations at the onset of labour; these form the basis of this Focus Group report. The enquiries had excluded congenital malformations and babies weighing less than 1.5kg, thus the findings relate primarily to the contributions of birth asphyxia and trauma to the cause of death.

A request was made to the relevant Regions for a copy of the anonymised medical records. Of the 56 cases, there were 51 full sets of notes available and the remaining five cases had reasonably detailed case summaries from which it was possible to obtain some data.

3.2.2 **Compiling a preliminary report - Standards Used**

The RCOG green top guideline[3] provided the standards against which the management of breech presentation in the 56 cases was judged. The data were collected using a detailed questionnaire, entered into a database and formed the basis of a preliminary report.

Part of the review comprised an assessment of the responses to cardiotocograph (CTG) traces. This was done by three midwives using the Nottingham City Hospital Intrapartum fetal monitoring guidelines[4] These are reproduced in Appendix 4. Each twenty minute section was classified as normal, suspicious or pathological as defined by FIGO[5] (Fédération Internationale de Gynécologie et d'Obstétrique). The times when action according to the guidelines should have been taken were noted for each trace. The case notes were then reviewed separately and a record was made of the times at which an appropriate action was initiated by staff in response to the CTG. The two sets of recordings for each case were compared to establish whether the response times met those defined by the Nottingham City Hospital guidelines.

A review of all the postmortem reports was undertaken by a perinatal pathologist.

3.2.3   **Formulating the recommendations - Multi-disciplinary group**
The preliminary report was circulated to a multi-disciplinary focus group, whose objective was to formulate recommendations for good practice in the management of breech presentation based on the findings of the preliminary report. The focus group was composed of obstetricians, midwives, paediatricians, specialist registrars, a public health specialist, a perinatal pathologist, a paramedic and lay members.

3.3   **THE FINDINGS**
There were 24 (43%) primipara and 32 (57%) multipara mothers.

Gestation and birthweight
The gestational age and birth weight distribution of the 55 babies at delivery are shown in Figure 3.1. There was 1 concealed pregnancy with no details. Just under half (43%) were preterm (less than 37 weeks gestation), but most of these delivered between 33 and 36 weeks. There were 5 babies on or below the 5th centile of birthweight as defined by the Northern region[6].

Figure 3.1 Gestational age and birth weight distribution at delivery

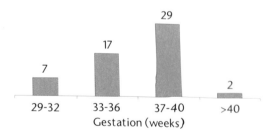

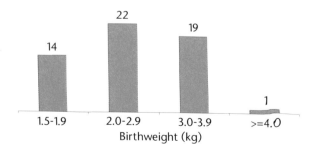

Breech Categories

The breech presentations were categorised as:

I   known prior to labour with delivery at 37 weeks or later (14)
II   unanticipated and recognised in labour in hospital (32)
III   delivering at home or in transit (11)

Figure 3.2 Breech categories

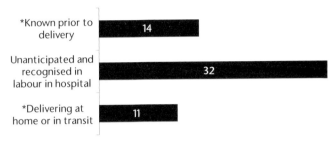

*1 of these babies falls into both categories

I: Breech presentation known prior to labour with delivery at 37 weeks or later (14 cases)

Assessment of the mother and baby at term involves discussion of the advantages and disadvantages of the various alternatives. This includes elective Caesarean section, external cephalic version (ECV) and trial of vaginal breech delivery. Just over half (8) of the notes recorded such a discussion.

Most (12) had plans generally made by the consultant for delivery (10 for vaginal delivery, 2 for Elective LSCS). Few plans mentioned fetal size and little use was made of ultrasound in the assessment.

External cephalic version was offered and attempted in 4 cases (3 at term, and 1 at 35 weeks). In at least one case the General Practitioner undertook this manoeuvre at a significant distance from a unit with suitable facilities for delivery. In two there was no plan for delivery following the attempted ECV. One was admitted at 39 weeks (2 weeks after ECV), with an antepartum haemorrhage and cord prolapse. In the other case, it was assumed that the woman would have a vaginal delivery when admitted in labour. The intrapartum management is described in Section 3.4.

II: Unanticipated breech presentation recognised in labour in hospital (32 cases)

This group comprised those in which the baby was first recognised to be breech during the course of labour (14 at term, 8 preterm) and those where the baby had been known to be breech antenatally but went into preterm labour (10). Half of these cases laboured in 'day time' hours, between 8.00 am and 6.00 pm. A consultant was informed of the admission prior to delivery in under half the cases (15). The intrapartum management is covered in Section 3.4

III: Breech presentation delivering unexpectedly at home or in transit (11 cases)

Of the 11 cases which delivered outside hospital, 6 were preterm, 4 were 40 weeks, and in one case the gestation was not known due to a concealed pregnancy.

Six of the babies were already delivering by the time a health professional attended and the actions taken in these circumstances were generally prompt and appropriate.

Paramedics or ambulance staff were often the first professionals at the scene of delivery at home or in transit. There were 7 cases where the paramedics were present for all or part of the delivery, or arrived shortly afterwards. A midwife was involved in 3 cases, one where she was present at the delivery, one where she arrived to find the woman had delivered half the body unattended, and the other where she arrived to assist the paramedic with the delivery of the head. In one case, a registrar from the obstetric flying squad took over from a husband delivering his wife at home.

Problems encountered at home included 6 cases where there was delay in delivery of the body and/or head. The longest documented body/head delivery interval in this group was 32 minutes.

Other problems included a cord prolapse in a planned home delivery thought to be cephalic until a breech presentation was found in the second stage of labour.

3.4	**INTRAPARTUM MANAGEMENT IN HOSPITAL**

Forty-five babies delivered in hospital, 20 of which were seriously compromised on admission. The reason for compromise included: bradycardia or absent FH (10); cord prolapse (5); significant APH (4) and cervical entrapment (1).

It is notable that nearly all (15/17) mothers in the unanticipated and uncompromised group were admitted at an early stage of labour with cervical dilatation of 4cm or less. Recognition of the correct presentation in this group was often late, with 4 diagnosed at full dilatation. There was no mention of the use of ultrasound in labour. The most senior person assessing the case in labour was usually the registrar. There were 5 cases where the most senior assessment was given by a senior house officer (SHO) (Figure 3.3).

Figure 3.3 Most senior person assessing the labour

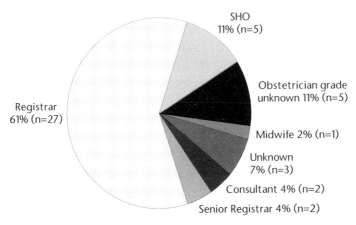

SHO
11% (n=5)

Obstetrician grade
unknown 11% (n=5)

Midwife 2% (n=1)

Unknown
7% (n=3)

Consultant 4% (n=2)

Senior Registrar 4% (n=2)

Registrar
61% (n=27)

Epidural anaesthesia was used in 15 cases. Labour was induced on 9 occasions.

Approximately a third (14/45) of labours were augmented. Frequently (6) syntocinon was commenced late in the 1st/2nd stage in multiparae. For cases with CTG traces available, definite abnormalities at the time of commencing syntocinon were present in at least half (7).

Para 2, admitted at 40+ weeks draining pinkish liquor not in established labour. Presentation thought to be cephalic. On VE, cervix 2-3 cms dilated, breech diagnosed. Confirmed by registrar, and decision made for trial of labour, epidural sited. CTG became suspicious but this was not recognised. Cervical dilatation arrested at 8 cm and after review by the registrar, syntocinon was commenced. CTG became pathological at full dilatation, no action was taken, commenced pushing an hour later. An assisted breech delivery was performed 80 minutes later. Baby born with Apgars of 0+0. Resuscitation abandoned after an hour.

3.4.1   **Intrapartum fetal surveillance**
There were 43 cases where some form of fetal monitoring was used (Table 3.1). There was no fetal blood sampling in any of the labours.

Table 3.1 Type of fetal monitoring used

Fetal monitoring	Number of cases
Not possible to monitor	13*
Proceeded to immediate delivery	5
Intermittent auscultation	5
Intermittent auscultation and continuous electronic fetal monitoring	4
Continuous electronic fetal monitoring	29
Total	*56*

*Deliveries at home or in transit (10), intrauterine deaths on admission in labour (3)

There were 33 cases where electronic fetal monitoring was used, and of these 24 CTG traces were available for review. Two were of such poor quality that assessment was not possible. In the 9 cases where no trace was provided the documentation recorded abnormal traces during part or most of the labour. The assessment of the actions in response to the abnormalities is described in the method section (Section 3.2). In 7 of the 22 cases where the CTG was available the actions were within those outlined by the Nottingham City Hospital guidelines. However, there were delays in responses ranging from 30 to 600 minutes in the remaining 15 cases, 7 of which were greater than 2 hours. These delays generally (13) occurred in the first stage of labour and were due to a failure to recognise the abnormality (8) or to act appropriately (7). In general there was a failure to appreciate the urgency or severity of the situation.

The following is an excerpt from a case where there was a prolonged delay in appropriate response to an initially suspicious and subsequently pathological trace.

A para 0 with a known breech presentation was transferred to delivery suite following augmentation for spontaneous rupture of membranes. The cervix was 6 cm dilated, and there was thick meconium draining. An epidural was sited, and a fetal electrode (FE) applied. Some early decelerations were noted from a 160bpm baseline. 2hrs later a further VE was performed to re-apply the FSE, the cervix was found to be an anterior lip only, with the breech at the spines. Deep decelerations developed, the woman was reviewed by the registrar, who planned to return and re-assess in an hour. Deep decelerations continued over the next hour and the registrar was informed.

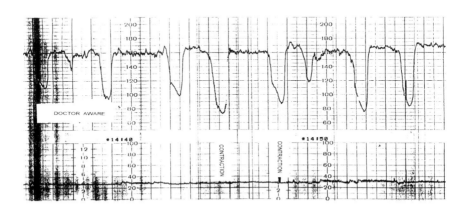

An hour later the registrar was busy and unable to re-assess. The FH fell to 60 bpm and did not recover. An emergency LSCS was performed the baby was born in poor condition and subsequently died.

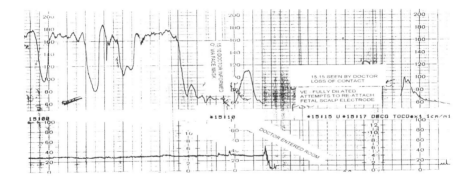

Intermittent auscultation (IA) was used in 5 cases, 4 in hospital. In two the death occurred in early labour on the antenatal ward. The other two hospital cases, were both known breech presentations and the midwives conducting the labours elected to use IA throughout labour. One had well documented recordings throughout the 1st stage of labour and the FH was noted after every contraction in the 2nd stage. The other case was poorly documented with infrequent recordings of the FH. The fifth case, where IA was used, was a planned delivery at home thought to be cephalic until a cord prolapse occurred and the breech was found at full dilatation.

3.4.2   Delivery in hospital
A third (15) were delivered by emergency Caesarean section. The decision-to-delivery interval in these cases was: within 30 minutes (9); between 36 - 49 minutes (4); and no information (2).

The registrar was generally the most senior person present at delivery (Figure 3.4).

Figure 3.4 Most senior person at delivery

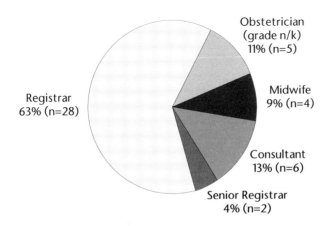

The vaginal delivery was documented as being difficult on 11 occasions. On reading the sequence of events there were other difficult deliveries, but there was discrepancy in the description. For instance, in one case the registrar documented an easy application of Neville Barnes forceps followed by easy delivery of the head over one contraction. However, the paediatric notes described the contrary ie. a very traumatic forceps delivery. The baby could not be resuscitated at birth and postmortem examination found fractures of the parietal bones, bilateral tentorial tears and massive subdural haemorrhage.

The difficulties incurred were with the after-coming head (6), cervical entrapment (4) and one with a problem with cord entanglement. Most (7), of these difficult deliveries had evidence of fetal compromise prior to delivery, rendering the fetus less able to withstand any additional asphyxial insult during delivery.

3.5   **BABY DETAILS**

3.5.1   **Condition at birth**
Half (28) of the cases had an Apgar of 0 at 5 minutes. A cord pH was taken in only 8 out of possible 45 cases.

3.5.2   **Resuscitation**
Excluding those deliveries which occurred outside the hospital, a paediatrician was present at delivery in 33 cases. The first paediatrician to attend was the SHO (15 cases), the registrar (9 cases), and the consultant (2 cases). There were 7 cases where the grade of the paediatrician was unclear from the notes. Of the 8 cases where a paediatrician was not present at delivery, 4 were cases where it was a known IUD, and in the other 4 cases the paediatrician was called prior to delivery, but did not arrive in time.

Neonatal resuscitation was attempted in 47 cases, and was considered to be adequate in 32 of these. There were 6 cases where there was insufficient documentation to comment on the adequacy of the resuscitation.

Some examples taken from the notes of the inadequacies in resuscitation are listed below:

'Midwife only able to administer funnel oxygen when called to unplanned home birth. No bag and mask available to enable adequate attempt at resuscitation.'

'SHO unable to intubate. Obstetric registrar and anaesthetist also failed. Baby finally intubated at 8 minutes of age by Consultant paediatrician.'

'Three attempts at intubation by paediatric SHO and anaesthetist. Paediatric registrar called, but not crash bleeped and took 10 minutes to arrive.'

'Took paediatrician 10 minutes to arrive. Obstetric registrar resuscitated and intubated baby until paediatrician arrived.'

'Paramedics resuscitated as best they could, but baby transferred to wrong hospital and by the time they arrived at correct unit, baby was severely hypothermic and hypoxic.'

3.6   **PATHOLOGY**

The examination of an infant who dies after vaginal breech delivery is important, as there is always the suspicion that trauma during delivery may have been a factor in the death. This can only be proven by a carefully performed postmortem, undertaken by a pathologist who is aware of the potential problems, since special techniques are required for reliable identification.

In the 41 babies delivering vaginally, postmortem had been carried out in 28, and 21 reports were available for review, 1 of which was provisional. For each report a 'breech score' of 0 to 4 was generated on the presence or absence of the following features:

- Occipital osteodiastasis (dislocation of the squamous occipital bone)
- Cervical spinal cord injury
- Dural tear
- X rays (lateral skull and whole body) undertaken to confirm or exclude fractures.

Assessment of 'breech related' pathology was relevant to 17 cases (three intrapartum stillbirths and one incomplete report were excluded). There were only 4 postmortem reports where all features were commented on (Table 3.2).

Dural tear was the feature most commonly commented on (10), followed by X-ray findings (9), and occipital bone (7) and cervical spinal cord (7) the least likely.

Table 3.2 Breech score of the postmortem report in the 17 cases with vaginal delivery.

Breech Score	Number of cases
4	4
3	3
2	2
1	3
0	5

The cause of death on the report was also reviewed to determine whether it was consistent with the clinical events and the pathological findings.

In three cases the given cause of death was incompatible with the documented postmortem findings and/or the clinical details of the case, for example, cause of death given as 'prematurity' in an unresuscitable, well grown 28 week infant.

Birth trauma alone was the given cause of death at postmortem in 1 case, birth trauma with hypoxia was described in a further 2 cases. The reviewer agreed with the 3 cases of birth trauma but felt there was evidence of hypoxia in all 3 cases. In 1 further case, the reviewer found that the post mortem report clearly described cerebral injury although this was not given as a cause of death.

Intrapartum asphyxia appears to have been understated as a cause of death. It was the stated cause of death at postmortem in 7 cases, but the reviewer found it was probably a major factor in 4 cases where no cause was given and in 3 cases where the diagnosis was judged to be wrong (Table 3.3).

Table 3.3 Agreement between pathology reviewer and reported findings in the 21 postmortems reviewed.

Cause of death reviewer	Cause of death PM report
Trauma	No cause of death but describes severe cerebral injury
Trauma/hypoxia	Trauma
Trauma/hypoxia	Trauma/hypoxia
Trauma/hypoxia	Trauma/hypoxia
Hypoxia	No cause given
Hypoxia	No cause given
Hypoxia	No cause given
Hypoxia	No cause given
Hypoxia	Other - prematurity
Hypoxia	Other (IVH RDS prematurity)
Hypoxia	Other (stillbirth)
Hypoxia	Hypoxia (minor trauma, CH)
Hypoxia	Hypoxia
Hypoxia	Hypoxia
Hypoxia	Hypoxia
Hypoxia	Hypoxia
Infection	Not known
Infection	Missing (probably infection)
Insufficient information	No cause given
Insufficient information	Hypoxia

Details of pathology specifically related to breech delivery and cranial trauma was generally poor.

This review, once again, reinforces the importance of high quality perinatal pathology services. The rarity of deaths after breech delivery means that only in specialist centres, with referrals from a large population base, is the necessary expertise likely to be available.

3.7   DISCUSSION

Breech presentation is known to be associated with a higher perinatal mortality and morbidity due to prematurity, congenital malformations and birth asphyxia or trauma[1]. However, as this review excludes both congenital abnormalities and babies weighing less than 1.5kg, the lessons learnt are more relevant to the contribution of birth asphyxia or trauma.

Approximately half of the 56 deaths were compromised in labour prior to contact with health care professionals. A fifth of the deaths occurred at home or in transit to hospital.

Actions by health professionals outside hospital were generally both prompt, and appropriate once problems had been identified. However, the unexpected nature of the events highlights how important it is to have an explicit plan of action for dealing with an undiagnosed breech at home. If delivery is not imminent, arrangements for transfer should be made by whichever professional is present. Hospital staff must be forewarned of the transfer and the reasons for it. Staff of appropriate speciality and seniority should be available to meet the woman to decide on further management.

The undiagnosed breech was the largest category of deaths and is the group most at risk. Most mothers in this group were admitted in the early stages of labour but the diagnosis was often not made until late in the first stage. Whilst it is generally accepted that failure to diagnose a breech is not necessarily associated with poor practice, increased effort both antenatally and in labour would have altered the management and might subsequently have avoided the death. Very little use was made of ultrasound, either antenatally or during labour itself.

External cephalic version reduces the chance of Caesarean section but was offered infrequently, possibly reflecting the practice in 1994-1995. It is of concern that ECV was performed in a setting where the baby could not be monitored nor delivered rapidly should an acute complication arise. There were two occasions on which no plans had been made for delivery: both followed failed ECV attempts. This precluded choice between alternative options in advance of the labour.

The commonest cause of death for these 56 babies was hypoxia. This was clear from the clinical review and confirmed by the postmortem findings. The single and most avoidable factor was the suboptimal care given in labour rather than the conduct of the delivery itself. Mechanical difficulties as a sole cause of death was rare. However, inexperience at the time of delivery exacerbated the risk to an already hypoxic baby.

Amongst babies who were not compromised on admission in labour there was often delay in recognising or responding to CTG abnormalities, frequently of the order of several hours. These delays were rarely due to single individuals but were usually due to a failure to appreciate the urgency or severity of the situation by an obstetric team.

There was often no senior involvement during the labour, possibly reflecting the standards of service provision. The registrar was usually the most senior doctor involved; this group includes some very experienced doctors but in general they are in training. Consultants were only informed of the admission in half of the cases.

Less than a quarter of the postmortems included a systematic and comprehensive examination of factors relevant to the death of a breech baby born vaginally, implying a lack of awareness of the problems of vaginal breech delivery. For the purposes of later case review and possible litigation, recording the absence of a potentially important lesion is as important as recording its presence.

> **In summary, the assessments and decisions made by health professionals, during labour, in particular those regarding intrapartum fetal surveillance, were the critical factors in the avoidable deaths.**

3.8 **RECOMMENDATIONS**

3.8.1 **Intrapartum care - general**
In view of the significant contribution of delays in response to hypoxia in labour the recommendations made by CESDI (4th Annual Report) after review of intrapartum deaths are repeated. A baby presenting by the breech is no different in its need for good maternity care from any other baby, therefore every hospital offering intrapartum care should have the following in place for all babies regardless of presentation.

- A regular rolling update/training programme in the use of CTGs for all professionals involved in intrapartum care. Ideally this should be done at least six monthly. Detailed indications for the use of CTGs should be included.
- Simple guidelines on interpretations of CTGs (what is a normal baseline, what is normal baseline variation and what is a deceleration) and what is an acceptable quality of recording.
- Guidelines on management options if a CTG is abnormal. (The CTG is a screen for intrapartum hypoxia; if abnormal, the options are either to perform a fetal blood sample in the first stage of labour, or to expedite delivery if a fetal blood sample cannot be obtained or in the second stage of labour). These guidelines should include reference to concomitant use of Syntocinon or regional analgesia with an abnormal CTG.

- Guidelines on referral practices and lines of communication with an abnormal CTG.
- Guidelines on the maximum time it should take to expedite delivery on the basis of presumed or confirmed intrapartum fetal hypoxia.

In addition to the above, accurate dates and times should be recorded on all traces and there should be local protocols for the storage of intrapartum CTGs.

CESDI wishes to highlight that the Department of Health has commissioned a national guideline on the use and interpretation of fetal heart surveillance. This is scheduled for release in 2001.

3.8.2   **Specific recommendations to the conduct of a breech presentation**

Antenatal management

- A plan should be made by 37 weeks gestation following a discussion of options available between an experienced practitioner and the mother. If recognition of the breech presentation occurs after this gestation then a plan should be formulated and recorded as soon as possible.
- Increased effort should be made to diagnose presentation at 37 weeks for all women planning to deliver outside an obstetric unit.
- Assessment should include an estimate of fetal size in relation to the mother, and careful assessment of both fetal and maternal well-being.
- ECV should be offered from 37 weeks and only undertaken with facilities for emergency delivery. A skilled obstetrician should perform it.

Intrapartum management

- On admission, a clinical assessment in labour should be carried out by the most experienced practitioner available and a clear plan of action discussed with the parents and documented in the labour records.
- The consultant should be informed of a breech presentation in labour and review the management plans for the conduct of the labour.
- Augmentation with syntocinon should not be used in the presence of fetal compromise.
- The most experienced practitioner available should be present to conduct or supervise the delivery.
- A skilled practitioner should be present for resuscitation with a practitioner skilled in neonatal intubation readily available [7].

Undiagnosed breech at home

- There should be local protocols for managing an undiagnosed breech at home.

Training, skills and experience of the intrapartum attendant

- Not all professionals will have the opportunity for hands on experience therefore alternative approaches to training such as the ALSO[8] (Advanced Life Support in Obstetrics) and MOET[9] (Managing Obstetric Emergencies and Trauma) courses should be made available.

Pathology

- Intrapartum related deaths after breech delivery should be examined by a perinatal pathologist or a general pathologist with a special interest, since these are rare cases and the pathology is easily missed.

REFERENCES

1   Cheng M, Hannah M (1993) Breech delivery at term: a critical review of the literature. *Obstet Gynecol:* **82** 605-18

2   CESDI 4th Annual Report, 1997

3   Royal College of Obstetricians and Gynaecologists. The management of breech presentation. Guideline No 20, RCOG July 1999

4   The Nottingham City Hospital (NHS Trust). Intrapartum fetal monitoring guidelines. Nottingham City Hospital 1999.

5   Fédération Internationale de Gynécologie et d'Obstétrique (FIGO) Guidelines for the use of fetal monitoring. International Journal of Gynaecology and Obstsetrics 1987; **25**: 159-167.

6   Tin W, Wariyar UK, Hey E N on behalf of the Northern Neonatal Network. British Journal of Obstetrics and Gynaecology 1997; **104** 180-185

7   Royal College of Paediatrics and Child Health and Royal College of Obstetricians and Gynaecologists. Resuscitation of Babies at Birth. London, BMJ Publishing Group, 1997

8   Kennedy J The Manet (Maternal and Neonatal Emergencies Training) Project, 47-49. London: Department of Health, 1997

9   Johanson R, Cox C et al Managing obstetric emergencies and trauma (MOET): Structured skills training using models and reality-based scenarios. The Obstetrician & Gynaecologist 1999 **1** No 2, 46-52.

ACKNOWLEDGEMENTS

Authors:
Mrs Cathy Winter, Midwife, CESDI
Mr Phillip Savage, Consultant Obstetrician and Gynaecologist, Southmead Hospital
Ms Joy Lawrence, Data Analyst, CESDI
Dr Phillip Cox, Senior Lecturer in Perinatal Pathology, Imperial College School of Medicine
Dr Mary Macintosh, Director, CESDI
Mrs Sian Warriner, Midwife, CESDI

With thanks to:
Ms Rosemary Buckley, Nottingham and Ms Tessa Mitchell, Birmingham for reviewing all CTG traces.

Members of the multidisciplinary panel

Ms Rosemary Buckley	Midwife, Nottingham City Hospital
Dr Jean Chapple	Public Health Consultant, Kensington Chelsea & Westminster Health Authority
Ms Mary Cronk	Midwife
Mr David Davies	Obstetrician, Hampshire
Mr Ed Dornan	Obstetrician (SpR), Homerton Hospital, London
Ms Jane Evans	Midwife, Lancashire
Mrs Marion Grant	Physiotherapist, Congleton Hospital
Dr Marion Hall	Obstetrician, Aberdeen Maternity Hospital
Mr Stephen Hines	Paramedic, London Ambulance Service
Dr Iona Jeffrey	Pathologist, St George's Hospital, London
Mr Tony Kelly	Obstetrician (SpR), Clinical Effectiveness Support Unit, RCOG
Dr C Burnett Lunan	Obstetrician, Glasgow
Ms Norah Malone	Midwife, Liverpool
Ms Tessa Mitchell	Midwife, Birmingham
Mrs Mary Newburn	National Childbirth Trust, London
Miss Zoe Penn	Obstetrician, Chelsea & Westminster Hospital
Dr Sunit Rane	Obstetrician (SpR) Hampshire
Dr Janet Rennie	Paediatrician, Kings College Hospital
Ms Brenda Van Der Kooy	Midwife
Mr Stephen Walkinshaw	Obstetrician, Liverpool Women's Hospital

4

FOCUS GROUP - OBSTETRIC ANAESTHESIA - DELAYS AND COMPLICATIONS

4.1   BACKGROUND

The safety of modern obstetric care is based on teamwork. In obstetric units today many women receive anaesthetic procedures, including regional analgesia in labour. The anaesthetist is a key member of the multidisciplinary perinatal management team.

The death of a baby as a result of an event in labour is a rare (approximately 1 in 1500 deliveries) and traumatic circumstance. Although it is unusual for the anaesthetic care to contribute directly to the death of the baby, these labours are often complicated and there may be circumstances where there are significant difficulties in the provision of the anaesthesia.

This year CESDI in collaboration with the Obstetric Anaesthetists' Association (OAA) reviewed the 1994-95 enquiries on intrapartum related deaths to identify suitable cases for a Focus Group Report. The aim of the Focus Group was to highlight issues of concern regarding serious complications and delays in the provision of the anaesthesia and to make recommendations for future practice.

4.2   METHOD

4.2.1   Identification of cases

CESDI reported the findings of the enquiries on all (873) normally formed babies weighing 1.5kg or over at birth who died as a result of an intrapartum event in 1994-1995 (4th Annual Report).

All enquiry cases with a comment attributed to an anaesthetist were identified. In addition the summaries provided by the panels were reviewed for incidents involving the anaesthetist. This identified 54 cases. A request was made to the relevant Regions for a copy of the corresponding anonymised medical records. These were reviewed by the authors and it was determined that in 29 cases the involvement of the anaesthetist was either after the death of the fetus or so peripheral to the event as to be not relevant. This left a total of 25 cases. In 20 of these full notes were available but in 5 cases only a summary of the events was available. This report is based upon these 25 cases. The term 'delay' refers to any delay involved in the delivery of the baby rather than a 'delay' in the widely accepted guideline of 30 minutes between decision-to-deliver (D-D) interval.

The data were collected using a detailed questionnaire. These were reviewed by the authors who compiled a preliminary report.

It has to be acknowledged that there were limitations to the identification of all relevant anaesthetic incidents. The enquiries in

1994/95 did not always have an anaesthetist on the panel and so there may be an under-estimate of such circumstances. The role of anaesthetists in subsequent CESDI panels is under review though the lessons that can be drawn from these cases are most important.

4.2.2 **Formulating the recommendations - Multidisciplinary group**
The preliminary report was circulated to a multidisciplinary Focus Group, whose objective was to formulate recommendations for good practice in the provision of the anaesthetic management based on the findings of the preliminary report. In addition to the authors, the Focus Group was composed of anaesthetists, operating department assistants, obstetricians, midwives, paediatricians, a public health consultant, and lay members.

4.3. **THE FINDINGS - 25 ANAESTHETIC INCIDENTS**
The type of anaesthetic administered involved general (19), spinal (3) and epidural (3) anaesthesia. There were no maternal deaths. The cases fell into three categories:

- Serious complications related to giving an anaesthetic (4 cases)
- Delays with personnel (11 cases)
- Delay in the provision of anaesthesia once the anaesthetist was available - either regional or general (10 cases).

4.3.1 **Issues directly related to giving an anaesthetic (4 cases)**
There were four cases, which were associated with a serious complication as a result of giving a general anaesthetic. These comprised two episodes of anaphylaxis, one of which led directly to the death of the baby; one failed intubation and one difficult intubation.

Grade III anaphylaxis
This woman was booked for an elective Caesarean section for a breech presentation. The pre-operative anaesthetic assessment was unremarkable. There was no documentation as to whether regional anaesthesia was discussed. The choice of a general anaesthetic was maternal because of her anxieties regarding 'awareness'. The grade of the anaesthetist was not documented. Anaesthesia was induced with thiopentone 425mg and suxamethonium after which the trachea was intubated. The haemoglobin oxygen saturation (SpO₂) fell to 67% and the lungs were difficult to ventilate. It was assumed that the woman had developed an anaphylactic reaction to either thiopentone or suxamethonium and hydrocortisone and chlorpheniramine were administered and the patient was woken up. SpO₂ remained below 80% for about 40 minutes. Spinal anaesthesia was administered and the baby delivered 49 minutes after the start of anaesthesia. Epinephrine (adrenaline) was administered to the mother after the delivery. The notes indicate that earlier epinephrine was not given in the belief that placental perfusion would be compromised.

Bronchospasm and hypoxia
This woman was booked for an elective Caesarean section. She had had a previous Caesarean section and the baby was thought to be growth restricted. It was noted in the pre-operative assessment that she was a smoker, she was asthmatic and had had bronchospasm during her general anaesthetic for her last Caesarean section. There was no documentation of any discussion about the risks and benefits of general and regional anaesthesia.
The consultant anaesthetist induced anaesthesia with thiopentone (?dose) and suxamethonium 100mgs and the trachea was intubated easily. The patient developed severe bronchospasm hypotension and generalised erythema. Oxygen 100% was administered and the SpO₂ was around 60%. Aminophylline and epinephrine were administered with an improvement in the mother's condition. Anaesthesia commenced at 12.00hrs and the baby was delivered at 12.38hrs.

Failed intubation
This woman had a placental abruption with severe fetal distress and was administered a general anaesthetic. At laryngoscopy the larynx could be visualised (grade 3) but there was laryngeal oedema which made intubation, even with the aid of a bougie, impossible. Good SpO₂ was maintained throughout and the airway managed with a laryngeal mask airway. At delivery of the baby there was a large retroplacental clot.

Difficult intubation.
This woman presented with severe fetal distress, the decision to deliver by Caesarean section was made and anaesthesia was commenced 5 minutes later. A general anaesthetic was administered with thiopentone 400 plus 400mg and two doses of suxamethonium 100mg and atropine 0.6mg x 2. The documentation was poor and it was unclear whether there was any visualisation of the glottis or whether the larynx was intubated at any time. The patient was ventilated with a mask and airway however, there was a significant period when the SpO₂ was around 60-70%. The decision to delivery interval was 23 minutes. There was a major placental abruption and the mother was transferred to the intensive care unit after delivery. It was not clear whether the need for intensive care was as a result of the intubation difficulties or the abruption. Hydrocortisone was administered suggesting concern that the mother may have aspirated.

4.3.2 Delays with personnel (11 cases)

There were 11 cases in which there was delay getting appropriate staff. The times of day involved had no particular pattern and were randomly distributed throughout the 24 hours.

Waiting for an anaesthetist accounted for 6 cases. Waiting for skilled assistance for the anaesthetist accounted for 4 cases. Waiting for a back-up delivery team accounted for 1 case. The delivery suite was so busy that the anaesthetist was involved with several other women and delays were also incurred by a lack of availability of an obstetrician.

A description of the delays incurred and the decision-to-delivery interval (D-D) is given in Table 4.1.

Two examples include:

A decision was made for immediate Caesarean section in a woman with persistent abnormality of the CTG. All personnel, except the anaesthetist, were present in theatre within 7 minutes. The duty obstetric anaesthetist was delayed elsewhere outside the maternity unit. However, the second anaesthetist did not arrive for a further 21 minutes. Unfortunately, this infant was stillborn and a diagnosis of placental abruption was made.

Following a decision to perform a Caesarean section for fetal distress the patient was moved to theatre. However, 15 minutes later, because neither the anaesthetist nor the skilled anaesthetic assistant had arrived, the patient was returned to the ward. A further 9 minutes elapsed before the patient was taken back to theatre, the baby was delivered stillborn 25 minutes later.

Table 4.1 Anaesthetic staff delays

D-D interval (minutes)	Reason given for delay
27	First ODA (Operating Department Assistant) busy with another case. Called second ODA from home, but eventually assisted by another doctor
37	Duty anaesthetist attending another Caesarean section so consultant anaesthetist had to be called from home
44	20 minute delay in the arrival of anaesthetist
48	Obstetric anaesthetist held up in Intensive Therapy Unit and main theatre with "overwhelming workload". Anaesthetist from general theatre sent to help
49	Patient and staff in theatre within 15 minutes of decision-to-deliver but no ODA. Patient taken back to ward and returned to theatre 10 minutes later. Not known whether or when ODA arrived
57	25 minutes getting woman to theatre, then further 22 minutes waiting for ODA
60	13 minute delay waiting for anaesthetist to arrive and a further 47 minutes to delivery. Reason for delay not documented

D-D interval (minutes)	Reason given for delay
60	First recordings by anaesthetist appear 25 minutes after patient arrival in theatre - reason for delay not documented
68	ODA not available and after a 10 minute wait, decided to call a second anaesthetist to assist instead
80	30 minutes from decision-to-deliver to arrival in theatre; 30 minutes wait for consultant anaesthetist and a further 20 minutes to deliver. No reason documented for delays
191	Very busy delivery suite with at least 2 other women requiring Caesarean section. Midwife suggested opening a second theatre but this was rejected by medical staff

4.3.3 **Delay in the provision of anaesthesia once the anaesthetist was available (10 cases)**

Regional anaesthesia was used in all of these cases. General anaesthesia was resorted to in 4 situations (3 following failed spinals with D-D intervals of 30, 32 and 40 minutes respectively) and 1 after failed epidural top-up with D-D interval of 38 minutes.

In the remaining six the longest delays involved top-ups of in situ epidurals with 3 cases having D-D intervals of 71, 80 and 85 minutes respectively. There were three successful spinals with D-D intervals 33, 35 and 65 minutes. (Figure 4.1)

It had been recognised antenatally that a woman with severe asthma had an increased risk from general anaesthesia. The consultant anaesthetist had written a full plan for analgesia and anaesthesia for delivery. An epidural in situ was topped-up to provide anaesthesia for Caesarean section because of delay in the progression of labour and fetal bradycardia. The top-up of 10 ml of 0.5% bupivacaine given was insufficient for anaesthesia. The anaesthetist was unhappy to give a general anaesthetic without the consultant, which resulted in delay.

Figure 4.1 Delays in administering anaesthetic (GA = General Anaesthesia)

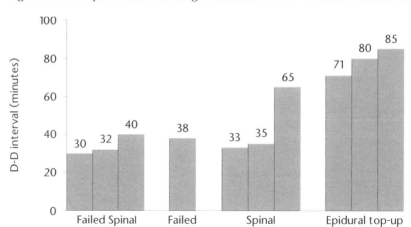

4.3.4 Documentation issues

The anaesthetic record was not available for review in 9/25 (36%) of the cases. However, the two important times, decision for Caesarean section and time of delivery were well documented, enabling the D-D interval to be calculated in every case.

For every case where there was a delay of more than 38 minutes in administering the anaesthetic, there was no reason for the delay documented in the notes, which made interpretation of this information unsatisfactory.

Where there were staff delays, it was difficult to determine when the absent anaesthetist or ODA actually arrived in theatre as these times were not generally documented. The presence or absence of an ODA at delivery was particularly badly documented. The member of staff involved and the reason for their delay was documented in 6 out of the 11 cases.

4. 4 DISCUSSION

The approach used to identify these cases is likely to have under-ascertained the number of serious complications and delays in anaesthetic involvement in the intrapartum related death enquiries. This was due to the lack of an anaesthetist and a failure to systematically record such events at the panel assessment. However, the lessons that can be drawn from these cases remain important.

4.4.1 Staffing and organisational factors

The largest contributing factor to the deaths of the babies was delay in assembling the delivery team. Unexpected emergency situations requiring the immediate presence of skilled staff are unavoidable, but it is important to ensure that the recommended minimum staffing levels are met by each Trust. Guidance on obstetric anaesthetic services has been set by the Association of Anaesthetists of Great Britain and Ireland and Obstetric Anaesthetists' Association 1998[1], and the Royal College of Anaesthetists in 1999[2].

These include that a resident anaesthetist should be provided for all consultant units. They should have more than one years anaesthetic experience, be immediately available and have their competency assessed by a consultant anaesthetist. Where a resident anaesthetist is not provided in smaller consultant units, a non-resident anaesthetist must be available to ensure that a delivery within 30 minutes of the decision would be possible. Trained dedicated assistance must be available for the anaesthetist at all times[3].

In the CESDI study nearly all staffing delays related to the primary on-call team. Failures to call personnel in good time led to unnecessary delays in addition to lack of immediate availability. Often the skilled anaesthetic assistance may have had a multiplicity of duties leading to uncertainties regarding his/her priorities.

4.4.2   **Communicating the degree of urgency**
There is no standard classification of degrees of urgency for the need to deliver a baby. This is partly due to the widely varying clinical circumstances, and also to the difficulty of predicting the long-term outcome of fetal hypoxia. There is a generally agreed recommendation[1,4,5] that emergency Caesarean section should be achieved within 30 minutes of the decision to operate. However, this is a pragmatic rather than 'evidence' based rule. Furthermore, rapid and precise communication between professionals as to the degree of urgency is essential. The lack of a systematic approach undoubtedly contributes to avoidable delays. Promising initiatives in this area should be developed and evaluated[6].

4.4.3   **Choice of anaesthesia for urgent Caesarean section**
General anaesthesia has the perceived advantage over spinal anaesthesia of rapid induction with little variation between anaesthetists or patients. However, it is associated with increased risks to the mother which at times may be life threatening and result in serious morbidity. Experience and skill are needed to achieve a satisfactory balance of maternal and fetal risk in urgent situations. Alternative approaches such as topping-up an existing epidural are only appropriate if they are rapidly effective.

In the studies reported here, general anaesthesia was used in most cases; a quarter of these represented a change from the initial procedure. Delays due to a lack of awareness of the passage of time were common. The delivery team, as well as the anaesthetist, are responsible for safe and rapid delivery. Reluctance by obstetricians and midwives to 'interrupt' anaesthetists, particularly if they are having difficulties, may contribute.

Hesitation in deciding to administer general anaesthesia occurred in some cases, particularly where there were serious risk factors for the mother and adequate senior help was not immediately available.

4.4.4   **Transfer to the theatre**
The best way to monitor the fetus during emergency transfer to the theatre is uncertain. The fetal heart should be confirmed prior to

delivery, but the extent to which this is done is a compromise between the need for immediate delivery and the need to be informed of the fetal condition. This is especially relevant if there is an unanticipated delay following the decision to deliver. It is important not to delay delivery by 'superfluous monitoring'.

4.4.5 **General anaesthesia and anaphylaxis**
Administration of a general anaesthetic will always carry the risk of anaphylaxis or severe bronchospasm. This risk is greater than with regional analgesia and is a valid reason for discussing all options for the anaesthetic technique.

This occurred in two instances, leading to delay in delivery while the mother's condition was stabilised. But these delays were unnecessary: rapid delivery has no deleterious effect on the ongoing treatment and resuscitation of the mother, and may even aid resuscitation of the mother [7,8].

Epinephrine is the drug of choice in the treatment of anaphylaxis, even in pregnancy. In the low cardiac output state of severe anaphylaxis, epinephrine is likely to improve rather than to reduce utero-placental blood flow.

4.4.6 **Auditing and measuring performance**
Demonstrating effective performance is an increasingly important requirement, in particular for external hospital reviews. Adherence to 'the 30 minute rule' is a level 3 requirement for the Clinical Negligence Scheme for Trusts (CNST)[9]. This standard was not met in 19 cases, though the feasibility of meeting this standard for all emergency deliveries has been questioned[4,5]. In the future, all trusts may be required to audit this standard, and this process will provide important benchmarking information which will address the issue of feasibility.

Decision to delivery time does not in itself identify which particular aspects of care contribute to the delay. Additional data is needed, especially when the patient reaches the operating theatre and when the anaesthetist is informed. This would distinguish between delays due to transfer to theatre, non-availability of the anaesthetist and problems in administering the anaesthetic.

4.5 **RECOMMENDATIONS**

4.5.1 **Staffing and organisational factors**
- The recommended staffing levels, as set out in Guidelines on Obstetric Anaesthetic Services [1,3] and Guidelines for the provision of Anaesthetic Services [2] should be met.

- A resident anaesthetist should be provided for all consultant units and should be immediately available. They should have more than one year of anaesthetic experience and have had their competence in obstetric anaesthesia assessed by a consultant anaesthetist. In smaller consultant units, a non-resident anaesthetist must be available to ensure delivery within 30 minutes of the decision.

- Trained dedicated assistance must be available for the anaesthetist at all times.

- A list of names of staff and methods of urgent contact should be available at all times on the delivery suite.

- There should be specific detailed arrangements if the primary contact is unavailable.

4.5.2   **Communicating the degree of urgency**
- There is an urgent need for a clear classification of the urgency of Caesarean section based on clinical scenarios. The classification should specify a target time and be recognised by professional bodies.

- There should be a clear verbal communication between all professionals as to the degree of urgency.   The obstetrician is responsible for initiating this process and local guidelines should be in place to effect it. The degree of urgency should be recorded in the notes.

4.5.3   **Choice of anaesthesia - antenatally**
- All pregnant women should be given clear information about the risks and benefits of general and regional anaesthesia for Caesarean section or other urgent delivery. An information leaflet would be helpful in disseminating this information in good time for women who were having a planned operative delivery.

- Women with significant risk factors for anaesthesia or analgesia should be assessed by an anaesthetist prior to delivery or labour. This can lead to a plan for delivery, which should include anaesthesia and analgesia and specify the grades of staff who should be involved and available at all times. A list of such factors should be provided in each unit.

4.5.4   **Choice of anaesthesia - urgent Caesarean section**
Experience and skill are needed to achieve a satisfactory balance between maternal and fetal risk in urgent situations. ALL pregnant women who have extant risk factors for anaesthesia, regional or general, should be assessed by an experienced obstetric anaesthetist during pregnancy, so that an anaesthesia management plan can be formulated and documented.

- If spinal anaesthesia is used in an urgent situation, repeated attempts are inadvisable in the absence of significant risk factors for general anaesthesia.

- On occasions it may be appropriate to top up an in situ epidural, though the urgency of the delivery requires that it must be rapidly effective. Epidurals should not be initiated in urgent situations.

- When top-up epidural anaesthesia is used, it should be commenced at the woman's bedside in order to reduce the time of transfer. The anaesthetist should accompany the woman to theatre. If the block is not satisfactory on reaching the theatre an alternative anaesthetic should be considered.

- General anaesthesia may be the preferred technique but there should be clear reasons for this choice as it is still associated with life threatening hazards.

4.5.5 **General anaesthesia and anaphylaxis or severe bronchospasm**
- Rapid delivery by Caesarean section is indicated in both the interests of the mother and fetus.

- All staff in maternity units should be aware of fetal and maternal resuscitation techniques and should maintain their skills with regular updating. Epinephrine is the drug treatment of choice for severe anaphylaxis[10].

4.5.6 **Auditing and measuring performance**
- Times should be routinely recorded and audited in all cases of emergency delivery. These should include the time at which the decision to deliver is made; the patient is in the operating theatre; and the time of delivery. The anaesthetist should document the time that s/he was informed of the decision to deliver, and when s/he was available. Reasons for delay should be documented.

- Benchmarking data on the decision-to-delivery (D-D) interval should be gathered to assess the feasibility of the widely accepted 30 minute rule.

- A high standard of record keeping should be encouraged by all levels of staff. Anaesthetists should be advised to make comprehensive, legible contemporaneous notes within the patients' records and not just rely on an anaesthetic chart. These notes may need to be made in retrospect.

REFERENCES

1. Guidelines for Obstetric Anaesthesia Services. Association of Anaesthetists of Great Britain and Ireland and Obstetric Anaesthetists' Association. London 1998.

2. Guidelines for the provision of Anaesthetic Services. The Royal College of Anaesthetists, July 1999

3. The Anaesthesia Team. Association of Anaesthetists of Great Britain and Ireland; London 1998.

4.   Tuffnell DJ, Wilkinson K (1998). Audit of time from decision to delivery for Caesarean Section. Royal College of Obstetricians and Gynaecologists, Audit in Obstetrics and Gynaecology: Achieving change with Audit. 24 Nov 1998.

5.   Dwyer JP (1999). Decision to delivery time in emergency caesarean section. Fourth International Scientific meeting of the Royal College of Obstetricians and Gynaecologists. Cape Town. 4-6 Oct 1999.

6.   Lucas DN, Yentis SM, Knsella SM, Holdcroft A, May AE, Wee M, Robinson PN. Development and evaluation of a new classification of urgency of Caesarean section. Journal of the Royal Society of Medicine (in press).

7.   Katz VL, Dotters DJ, Droegmueller W. Perimortem Caesarean delivery. Obstet Gynecol 1986; 68: 571-576

8.   Marx GF. Cardiopulmonary resuscitation of late-pregnant women. Anesthesiology 1986; 56: 156

9.   CNST Risk Management Standards. Nov 1999.

10. Kaplan PA. Allergy. 2nd Edition 1997. WB Saunders Co, Philadelphia. Chap 34, 571 - 572

ACKNOWLEDGEMENTS

Authors:
Dr Anne May, Anaesthetist, Leicester Royal Infirmary,
Dr John Crowhurst, Anaesthetist, Queen Charlotte's Hospital, London
Mr Derek Tuffnell, Obstetrician, Bradford Royal Infirmary
Dr Mary Macintosh, Director, CESDI (editorial contribution)

With thanks to
Dr Paul Howell, Anaesthetist, St Bartholomew's and Homerton Hospitals. London
Dr Elizabeth McGrady, Anaesthetist, Glasgow Royal Infirmary
Dr Tamara Madej, Anaesthetist, York District Hospital
Dr Michael Mitchell, Anaesthetist, Royal Cornwall Hospitals

MEMBERS OF THE MULTIDISCIPLINARY PANEL

Dr Summi Abdul	Obstetrician, Bradford Royal Infirmary
Mr Vince Argent	Obstetrician, Eastbourne DGH
Dr Samina Bharmal	Anaesthetist, Leicester Royal Infirmary
Dr Griselda Cooper	Anaesthetist, Queen Elizabeth Hospital, Birmingham
Dr Leslie Davidson	Perinatal Epidemiologist and Public Health Consultant Director, National Perinatal Epidemiology Unit
Ms Tina Delaney	Midwife, University of Wales, Cardiff

Dr Paul Howell	Anaesthetist, St Bartholomew's and Homerton Hospitals. London
Ms Dawn Jary	Secretary, Association of Operating Department Practioners (AODP)
Mr Bill Kilvington	Chairman, The Association of Operating Department Practitioners (AODP)
Mrs Lucy Lelliott	SANDS representative, Wiltshire
Mr Stephen Lindow	Obstetrician, Hull Maternity Hospital
Dr Mary Macintosh	CESDI - Director
Dr Elizabeth McGrady	Anaesthetist, Glasgow Royal Infirmary
Dr John McIntyre	Senior Lecturer in Child Health, Derbyshire Children's Hospital
Dr Tamara Madej	Anaesthetist, York District Hospital
Ms Stephanie Meakin	Midwife, Royal College of Midwives
Dr Michael Mitchell	Anaesthetist, Royal Cornwall Hospitals
Dr Phil Moore	Anaesthetist, Birmingham Women's Hospital
Dr Lynne Rogerson	Obstetrician, St James Hospital, Leeds
Prof. Nicholas Rutter	Paediatrician, Queens Medical Centre, Nottingham
Ms Shirley Smith	Midwife, Royal Free Hospital, London
Ms Gail Workmeister	Lay member, London

5

CARDIOTOCOGRAPH EDUCATION SURVEY

5.1 **INTRODUCTION**

Intrapartum related deaths represent 4.5% of deaths in the range covered by CESDI, that is, from 20 weeks' gestation until one year of life. In 1994-1995 there were 873 such deaths of babies weighing over 1.5 kg. In more than 75% of these cases there was evidence of suboptimal care such that alternative management 'might' (grade 2) or 'would reasonably be expected to' (grade 3) have made a difference to the outcome. More than half of the comments related to failures in the use and interpretation of cardiotocograph (CTG) tracings. CESDI therefore recommended that every hospital offering intrapartum care should have in place a regular rolling update/training programme in the use of CTGs for all professionals involved in intrapartum care (4th Annual Report).

The 5th and 6th Annual Reports also highlighted criticisms of CTG interpretation. In order to assess the degree to which the recommendations of the various Annual Reports have been acted upon, it was decided to conduct a survey of the provision of CTG education to midwives and obstetricians involved in intrapartum care. The study aimed to quantify the availability and scope of training. It did not address the effectiveness of such training in terms of changing clinical practice and/or affecting outcome.

5.2 **METHOD**

5.2.1 **Scope of study**

The scope of the study was to include all maternity units in England, Wales and Northern Ireland, including midwife-led units, independent birth centres and private maternity hospitals.

Establishing such a list with the corresponding names of the district tutors for obstetrics and heads of midwifery was not a straight forward process. This was due to the number of units being in an almost constant state of flux, with units merging or closing and Trusts changing names. The final list consisted of 226 District Tutors and 261 senior midwives/Heads of Midwifery. The greater number of midwives contacted is accounted for by low-risk units where obstetric staff are not routinely based.

5.2.2 **Design of questionnaire**

The questionnaire was limited to four sides of A4 to encourage completion (A summary of the questions covered can be found at the end of this chapter). The topics covered included availability of education, attendance of various grades, content of courses and teaching methods used, provision of study leave/funding for CTG education. The opportunity was also taken to ask a question concerning resuscitation skills training for midwives. Separate questionnaires were designed for midwives and for obstetricians, although there was a considerable overlap of questions. This reflected the different post-qualification training structures for midwives and for obstetricians.

The draft questionnaires were circulated to 4 midwives/midwife educators and 6 obstetricians for comment prior to piloting in 10 hospitals, each in a different Region. Two hospitals with 5000+ deliveries annually were chosen, 5 units with 2000-5000 deliveries and 3 units with 1000-2000 deliveries. One of the large units and one of the medium units were teaching hospitals. Only minor amendments were suggested.

5.2.3   **Main survey**
487 forms were sent out by post at the end of July 1999, each with a covering letter explaining the background to the survey. Notes were given on how to fill in the various sections of the form. A pre-paid business reply envelope was provided. Repeat forms were sent to non-responders. The data was entered on to two tables in a Microsoft ACCESS database.

5.3   **RESULTS**

5.3.1   **Response rate**
The response rates were 95% (245/257) from midwives and 85% (187/221) from obstetricians. Only one unit failed to produce a response from either the obstetric or the midwifery department. Most questions were answered by 95% of responders. The questions which were less well answered were those concerning attendance of staff at training. Where the denominator differs from the overall survey size, this is because some units did not answer particular questions.

5.3.2   **Characteristics of units**
The units were classified according to number of deliveries using the classification of consultant units used by the RCOG and RCM in their report Towards Safer Childbirth (1999)[1].

Small   A   up to 1000 deliveries
Medium B   between 1000 and 4000 deliveries
Large   C   greater than 4000 deliveries and/or tertiary referrals

Of the 261 responding units, 33 had fewer than 1000 deliveries in 1998. Units with 1001-2000 deliveries in that year comprised 20% of units. The majority (52%) of units had 2001-4000 deliveries in 1998. There were 3 units with 6000 deliveries or more per year (Figure 5.1).

Figure 5.1 Distribution of units according to number of deliveries

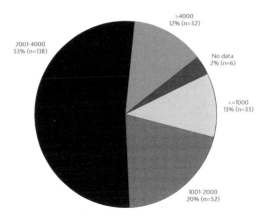

A consultant labour ward session is where the consultant is dedicated to the labour ward and has no other commitment. A session covers a half day. The number of Labour Ward consultant sessions covered per week ranged from none to 12.

The RCOG/RCM report recommended that all hospitals in category B have a target of 10 consultant sessions and all hospitals in category C target 24 hour consultant involvement with no other commitment.

The number of labour ward consultant sessions covered in medium and large units is shown in Figure 5.2:

Figure 5.2 Number of labour ward consultant sessions covered in medium and large units.

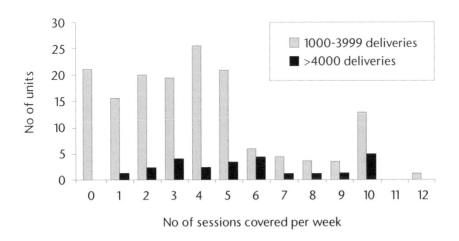

Heads of Midwifery were asked to provide information on the number of whole-time equivalent (WTE) midwives involved in intrapartum care, whether in the hospital or the community. The ratio of midwives (WTE) to number of deliveries ranged from 1:10 to 1:60. The lowest ratios were generally found in smaller, midwife-led units.

5.3.3 Provision/availability of training

The majority of responding units had CTG training available to their midwifery staff (96%, 233/244) and to their medical staff (98%, 181/185).

For the 9 units which did not have CTG training available for midwifery staff, the reasons given included the low-risk nature of the unit, with CTG not being used at all, and financial and time constraints. Six of the units had plans in place for training programmes to commence in either 1999 or 2000. In the 4 units where CTG training was not available to medical staff, this was stated to be because of time and resource constraints, particularly shortage of staff.

Training for midwives was provided locally in 91% (211/231) of units and elsewhere in 72% (166/231) of units. For obstetricians, the figures were 99% (177/179) and 14% (25/179) respectively.

Courses elsewhere included nationally-run fetal monitoring study days and the Advanced Life Support in Obstetrics (ALSO).

Amongst medical staff, CTG training was available to the majority. The Senior House Officers (SHOs) and Specialist Registrars (SpRs) were the junior grades most likely to have such training available. Staff grades and locums were less likely to have training available, as shown in Figure 5.3:

Figure 5.3 Availability of CTG training to obstetric staff (in 181 responding units)

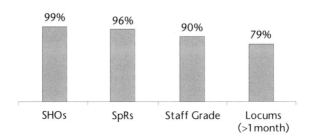

More than half of Regional training programmes for obstetricians included CTG training (62%, 115/186). These Regional training programmes are specifically for SpRs but were also open to SHOs (73 units), Consultants (22 units), Associate Specialists (6 units), and medical students (2 units).

5.3.4 Attendance patterns

Frequency of training recommended
The majority of units (80%, 185/230) recommended annual training for midwives, with 11% (26/230) recommending 6-monthly. The remaining units recommended other intervals, ranging from monthly to 2-yearly. For obstetricians, the majority recommended 6-monthly

training (54%, 100/187) and annually was recommended in 16% (30/187). For the remaining units intervals ranged from weekly to ad hoc.

Timing of training
For midwives, 56% (135/241) of units made CTG training available within 1-3 months of commencing a post. In the remaining 106 units, CTG training was made available later than this, or did not have any particular relationship to the timing of a post.

For obstetricians, the majority of units (90%, 166/185) made CTG training available to SHOs at induction or within the first month after appointment. For Specialist Registrars (SpRs), 31% (53/172) of units reported that CTG training was unrelated to the commencement of the post.

Compulsion
In 59% of units (133/225 responders) midwifery attendance at CTG training was compulsory, with monitoring being carried out mainly by managers and Supervisors of Midwives. Seven units expected individual midwives themselves to be responsible for making sure that they attended CTG training at appropriate intervals.

Attendance was compulsory for obstetricians in 71% (126/178) of units.

Documented evidence of training
88% (202/230) of responding units had documented evidence of midwifery attendance at CTG training. Attendance was frequently (90%, 198/221) recorded during an annual supervision interview; it was less often (64%, 96/151) recorded or discussed during an annual appraisal interview.

Half of the units (88/178) had documented evidence of medical attendance at training. It should be noted that a fifth of units did not respond to this question.

In units where information was available on the number of midwifery staff who attended training in the 12-month period concerned, attendance was reported as shown in Figure 5.4:

Figure 5.4 Midwifery staff attending training sessions - by grade (in 202 responding units)

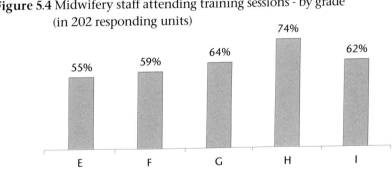

Grade of Midwife

For SHOs, most (82%, 86/105) responding units reported that over three quarters of staff had attended CTG training in the previous 12 months. However, nine units reported an attendance rate of less than 50%. Similarly for SpRs, most units (83%, 70/84) reported that over three quarters had attended, but eleven units had an attendance rate of less than 50%. Only a minority of units (12) provided information about locum attendance at CTG training; seven of the units reported 100% attendance. Of the 45 units which provided information on Staff Grade attendance at CTG training, 30 reported 100% attendance.

5.3.5   **Multidisciplinary training**
Attendance at CTG training was reported to be multidisciplinary in 79% (176/224) of responding units by midwives and in 81% (143/176) of units by obstetricians. There were 17 units where midwives answered yes to this question whereas the obstetrician answered no, and a further 18 where midwives said no and the obstetrician said yes. For 108 units both said yes, and for 10 units both said no. Joint attendance presented problems in a number of units. Comments made included:

-    *Junior doctors need prompting +++.*
-    *Very active participation from the consultants and midwives - very poor attendance from junior and registrar staff.*
-    *Midwives are invited but rarely come, except the most senior.*
-    *Difficulty experienced in getting midwives to attend regularly.*

5.3.6   **Training methods and settings**
Although the questionnaires aimed to separate informal from formal teaching, this was not easy to achieve in practice. There was considerable overlap, with case review meetings and CTG reviews, for instance, being included in either section.

Informal training consisted of small group or one-to-one training, perinatal mortality meetings or 'near miss'/interesting case meetings. These forms of teaching were used at between 77% and 90% of units. Other forms of informal training included Caesarean section reviews, CTG reviews, clinical case review meetings and risk management meetings.

Lectures were the most commonly used formal teaching method (88%, 203/231 midwifery responses, 79%, 138/175 medical responses). Computer-based interactive packages were being used in 29 units as reported by midwives, but in only 18 units according to the obstetricians. Practical exercises, implying active rather than passive learning, were also widely used (174 midwifery and 99 medical responses). Discussions and case reviews with problem-solving were additional components of formal training.

5.3.7   **Content of training courses**
The content of formal training showed broad similarities, as shown in Figure 5.5.

Figure 5.5 The content of CTG courses

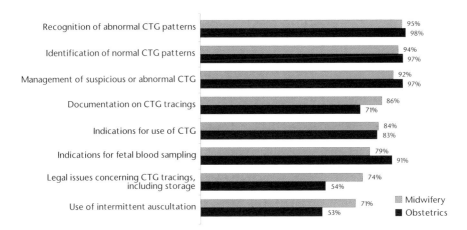

5.3.8 Evaluation of training

Evaluation of midwifery CTG training was undertaken in 39% (89/231) of responding units. This most often consisted of written evaluation forms at the end of training sessions.

For medical CTG training, there was evaluation of the training programme in only a small minority (11%, 19/175) of responding units. In the units where it did occur, it most commonly consisted of filling in evaluation forms and/or giving verbal feedback.

5.3.9 Costing/provision of study leave

For midwives, time off was usually granted for both in-house (89%) and formal (97%) CTG training courses. This was sometimes formally budgeted for through training or Human Resource budgets (132 units), but also through clinical area budgets (119 units). In 98 units, midwives were sometimes self-funded, particularly for formal external courses; in three units, self-funding was the only option for midwives attending formal training. In four units, funds were provided through special charitable trusts.

For obstetricians, the amount of time allocated to formal CTG training per trainee per 6 months varied enormously between units, ranging from 30 minutes to 48 hours. The majority of responding units reported a time allocation of 3 hours or less. SpRs had protected time to attend regional training sessions in most cases (94%, 168/178).

5.3.10 Resuscitation training

In 95% (226/238) of responding units all midwives were regularly attending neonatal resuscitation skills sessions. The most common frequency was annually. In only 7 units was the updating less often than annually. This question was not included in the obstetricians' questionnaire.

5.4   DISCUSSION

5.4.1   Staffing and organisation

The RCOG[1] has recommended that medium and large size units (category B and C) should target providing at least 40 hours (10 sessions) of consultant supervisory cover of labour ward. The larger units should have such cover at all times. This survey found that in 1998, 89% of units fell substantially short of this target. This shortage of consultant cover contributes to a lack of informal CTG training on the Labour Ward.

The survey found that the ratio of whole-time equivalent midwives to number of deliveries varied from 1:10 to 1:60. This suggests a wide variation in workload between units, although it is acknowledged that structures for providing midwifery services vary considerably, making direct comparison difficult. Many units (114/157) were still employing midwives on E grade. This is not in keeping with Department of Health guidance[2] that midwives giving the full range of care to women be employed on a minimum F grade.

5.4.2   Frequency of training

The frequency of training for CTG training was recommended annually by most units and falls short of the 6-monthly recommendations made by CESDI[3], the RCOG and RCM[1] and the Clinical Negligence Scheme for Trusts[4]. This was especially so for midwives compared with medical staff.

However, the term 'update' may be confusing as essentially in the context of CTG training the term 'refresher' may be more appropriate. The original recommendations were based on pragmatism in the absence of strong evidence. Six monthly is necessary to parallel the pattern of intakes of SHOs and ensure that they receive training before or very soon after taking up an appointment. In the majority of units there were difficulties co-ordinating the timing of training with the commencement of appointments. For midwives, an annual session may be adequate.

5.4.3   Range of personnel receiving training

It is noticeable that among midwives higher grades, including managers, have the highest attendance rate at CTG training. Staff of lower grades, who spend the highest proportion of their time giving clinical care, are the least likely to attend training. It is acknowledged that G or H grades may be providing clinical support to more junior midwives, and thus need to maintain their CTG interpretation skills. However, it is essential that the midwife providing direct care to the woman in labour is adequately trained in recognising and acting on abnormalities in the fetal heart rate. The reasons for a low attendance rate among junior midwives is not clear. Difficulties in releasing front-line staff were experienced for all grades. There may also be a particular problem in units with a large proportion of part-time staff.

Among medical staff, SHOs and SpRs were the most likely to have training offered to them, whereas staff grades and locums were the least likely. It is of concern that in a seventh of responding units fewer than 50% of SpRs had attended CTG training in the last 12 months. It is particularly important that these staff all receive training as they should usually be the first line of referral for midwives who have detected an abnormal CTG trace. Information about SpR attendance at CTG training was not available from a majority of units. It is therefore not possible to be sure what proportion of staff overall are actually being refreshed in their knowledge and skills in this important area.

5.4.4   **Style and content of training**
More than three quarters of the units reported that CTG training was multidisciplinary. This is appropriate, since the content of the training will be broadly similar for midwives and for obstetricians. Some barriers to multidisciplinary training were experienced, particularly the difficulty of releasing staff to attend training. Regional training programmes for obstetricians cover many other topics besides CTG interpretation and are therefore not relevant to midwives. This partly accounts for the segregation of training reported by some units.

It is notable that the topics least likely to be covered in formal CTG training were legal issues related to CTG tracings and the use of intermittent auscultation. Both these areas are of importance in clinical governance and risk management.

Although fewer than 10% of units had computer-based CTG education packages available, it seems likely that these will offer a practical solution to the problem of releasing front-line staff for study days. This applies particularly to midwives, with the ongoing shortage of staff making it difficult for them to attend training days. Computer-based programs can be readily accessed on most maternity units, and even a short session can be educationally useful. An additional advantage of such programs is that feedback can be incorporated into the training package.

5.4.5   **Documentation of attendance and evaluation of course**
Despite the high response rate overall for the survey, it was noticeable that the questions about number of staff attending training were poorly answered. Either the information was not available, or it was too difficult or time-consuming to retrieve.

There was little attempt to evaluate the courses, especially the medical training.

The availability of CTG education does not necessarily mean that any use is being made of it. Staff may never open the books that sit on a shelf in the Labour Ward sitting room, or may never log on to the computer program. This survey does not address the effectiveness of such training. Work in this area is limited although improved effectiveness of training in terms of increased core knowledge has been demonstrated using an interactive computer program compared with conventional methods[5].

5.4.6   **Costs of training**
Most formal CTG training is generally provided free to medical staff. The survey shows that many midwives are using both their own time and money to attend relevant training in many units.   It is inappropriate that this type of training should be left up to individuals rather than be considered essential by the Trust.   Paying for appropriate training for all relevant staff represents a far better use of funds than facing the increasing costs of litigation which may arise from instances of poor care[6].

5.5   **RECOMMENDATIONS**
- Trusts should be able to confirm that **all** staff involved in intrapartum care have received CTG training within the last year
- **All** staff providing intrapartum care should have access to CTG training.
- Trusts should ensure CTG training is available, and not expect midwives to fund it themselves.
- Interactive training packages should be made available on or near most Labour Wards.
- CTG training should include instruction on documentation on traces, and on storage[7].

It was very encouraging to receive such a high response rate to the survey questionnaires. It is possible that merely receiving a CESDI questionnaire on the subject of CTG education has stimulated action to remedy deficient education provision.   It is to be hoped that responses were honest rather than merely painting a favourable picture, and that training in this area will continue to improve.

REFERENCES
1   Towards Safer Childbirth, Minimum Standards for the Organisation of Labour Wards, Report of a Joint Working Party. Royal College of Obstetricians and Gynaecologists and Royal College of Midwives. February 1999

2   Changing patterns of maternity care: implications for pay and grading for midwives and for midwifery senior management posts. EL(95)77, Department of Health 1995

3   Confidential Enquiry into Stillbirths and Deaths in Infancy 4th Annual Report. Maternal and Child Health Research Consortium, London 1997

4   Clinical Negligence Scheme for Trusts.   Manual of Risk Management Standards. August 1999

5   Greene K. et al. The development and evaluation of a computer-based teaching package for intrapartum fetal monitoring. Unpublished article

6   Dyer, C.   NHS compensation bill set to soar.   Brit Med J 2000, 320:599

7   Symon, A. The importance of cardiotocographs. British Journal of Midwifery, Vol. 5, No 4, 1997

ACKNOWLEDGEMENTS

Author:
Mrs Niki Jakeman, Research Midwife, CESDI Secretariat

With thanks to:
The National Perinatal Epidemiology Unit, Oxford
Prof K Greene, Consultant Obstetrician, Derriford Hospital , Plymouth
All professional colleagues who kindly took the time to fill in and return the questionnaires

CTG EDUCATION SURVEY QUESTIONS

Unit characteristics
- **Number of births in 1998**
- Number of midwives, number of whole-time equivalents
- Number of obstetric consultant Labour Ward sessions covered
- Number of SHOs and SpRs involved in intrapartum care
- Number of other obstetric grades involved in intrapartum care
- **Presence of Risk Management Department**

Availability of CTG training
- **Is such training available to staff?**
- Does the regional training programme include sessions on CTG?
- Do SpRs have protected time to attend regional sessions?
- Do other obstetric staff attend regional sessions?
- Which grades of obstetric staff have CTG training available to them?
- **Where is CTG training provided - locally/elsewhere?**
- **What training resources are available on Labour Ward?**

Attendance patterns
- **Number of staff, listed in grades, who have attended CTG training in the last 12 months**
- **How often are staff recommended to attend training?**
- **How soon after appointment is CTG training made available?**
- **Is attendance compulsory?**
- **Is there documented evidence of attendance?**
- Who is responsible for monitoring attendance?
- Is attendance recorded at appraisal and/or supervision interviews?
- **Are sessions jointly attended by midwives and medical staff?**

Informal/in-house training
- **Teaching settings e.g. small group, 'near-miss' meetings, perinatal mortality meetings**
- Who leads the sessions?

Formal training/courses
- Teaching methods
- Content of training
- Who teaches the courses?
- How much time allotted to formal CTG training per trainee per 6 months?

Costing (midwifery questionnaire only)
- Is time off allocated for attendance at in-house CTG training?
- Is Study Leave granted for attendance at formal CTG courses?
- Whose budget pays for the cost of formal courses?

General
- **Is any evaluation of CTG training undertaken?**
- Do all midwives attend neonatal resuscitation skills sessions? How often?

Free text boxes for comments were included in each section of the questionnaires.

NOTE: Questions in **bold type** were included on both questionnaires. Questions in normal type were only on either the midwifery or the medical questionnaire.

6

SUDDEN UNEXPECTED DEATHS IN INFANCY - PATHOLOGY

6.1   **BACKGROUND**

Postmortem examination is a vital part of the investigation of sudden unexpected deaths in infancy (SUDI). It is essential for establishing the cause of death in those cases with recognisable illnesses such as pneumonia or meningitis (i.e. explained SUDI). Equally, a thorough postmortem examination is necessary to exclude natural or unnatural disease processes that might be responsible for death before Sudden Infant Death Syndrome (SIDS) can be given as the "cause" of death (i.e SIDS = Unexplained SUDI). Occasionally, postmortem examination demonstrates that an apparently natural death is due to injury.

The definition of SIDS stipulates that no cause of death is found after a "thorough" postmortem examination. There is broad agreement among pathologists with special experience in this field about the tests necessary to exclude common causes of unexpected death in infancy. However, although these investigations have been widely used in research studies, they have not been systematically evaluated in routine postmortem practice. The CESDI study provided a unique opportunity to evaluate their contribution to diagnosis and devise an evidence-based protocol.

6.2   **METHOD**

Pathologists were asked to carry out their postmortem examinations to a standard protocol[1] based on Royal College of Pathologists recommendations[2].

CESDI Regional Coordinators provided completed postmortem reports with hospital of origin and pathologists name removed. They also prepared an extra set of microscope slides.

Postmortem reports were each analysed by a regional pathology coordinator, without knowledge of the final conclusion reached by the local pathologist. A detailed protocol was used, revised after an initial pilot study, to ensure consistency.

From each report, the protocol involved: abstraction of basic demographic data; an assessment of the adequacy of clinical history to direct subsequent postmortem examination and ancillary investigations; a record of external and internal findings and investigations performed. In addition, the contribution of ancillary investigations to diagnosis was scored and the cause of death, together with the grade and discipline of the pathologist and the completeness of the postmortem report recorded.

The findings of the regional pathology coordinator were classified according to the Avon clinico-pathological classification[3]. Deaths were placed in one of three broad categories:

I.   no significant findings;
II. findings that may have contributed to ill-health and possibly to death;
III. findings that provide a full explanation for death.

Categories I and II constitute SIDS cases, category III non-SIDS.

Lastly, a comparison was made between the diagnosis made by the local pathologist, the regional co-ordinating pathologist and the diagnosis for each case after a local case discussion or confidential enquiry.

6.3   **RESULTS**
450 postmortem reports were received from 464 deaths which occurred during the period of study (97% ascertainment).

6.3.1   **Cause of death**
The cause of death was given as SIDS in 315 (70%) of cases, and non-SIDS in 135 (30%) of cases by the original pathologist. Using the Avon classification, the reviewer assigned 253 (56.2%) to group I (no pathological finding which contributed to death), 117 (26%) to group II (pathological findings which possibly or probably contributed to death and 80 (17.8%) to group III (death fully explained by the pathological findings). This revised approach gives 82% SIDS cases (Avon I + II) and 18% non-SIDS cases (Avon III).

6.3.2   **Pathologist**
Four per cent of examinations were carried out by trainees, 49% by consultant histopathologists, 32% by consultant paediatric pathologists and 14% by forensic pathologists.

Different subspecialists within pathology made different use of ancillary tests, most tests being undertaken by paediatric pathologists, fewest by forensic pathologists (Table 6.1).

Paediatric pathologists gave the cause of death as SIDS in 76% of cases, general pathologists in 70% and forensic pathologists in 59% of cases. (The case mix of the latter group included more suspected unnatural deaths.)

Table 6.1 Who includes what in their reports? Tests and conclusions reported by different pathology specialties

	General pathologists (% reported)	Paediatric pathologists (% reported)	Forensic pathologists (% reported)
Some history	95	92	89
X-ray report	53	69	47
Adequate histology	53	69	47
Frozen section report	33	70	8
Vitreous electrolytes	33	70	8
Blood culture report	61	86	19
CSF[1] bacteriology	61	77	23
Lung bacteriology	60	60	22
Lung virology	53	85	9
Toxicology	2	1.4	8
Final report	97	94	95
Non-SIDS diagnosis	30	24	41

[1]CSF = cerebrospinal fluid

6.3.3 Positive pathology tests in fully explained deaths

On review, 80 of the 450 cases were considered to have an underlying cause and be fully explained by findings (Table 6.2).

Histology was the single most useful investigation and was positive in 67% (Table 6.3). The contribution of the other tests to determining the cause of death is listed. The number of significant positive histological findings is given in Table 6.4.

When histology was positive, the respiratory tract was the most frequent site, closely followed by the central nervous system. Significant pathology in the lungs such as bronchiolitis could not be predicted reliably from macroscopic examination. In the original non-SIDS category, there was also over-interpretation of normal microscopic features of infant lung, such as peribronchial lymphoid aggregates, and some deaths were incorrectly attributed to aspiration of gastric contents.

Table 6.2 Cause of death in Avon group III cases

Organ system	Cause of death	No. of cases
Respiratory	Bronchiolitis	5
	Pneumonia	14
Central nervous system	Meningitis	4
	Encephalitis	2
	Trauma	10
	Vascular malformation	1
Cardiovascular	Myocarditis	4
	Cardiomyopathy	1
	Congenital	10
Gastro-intestinal	Intussusception	2
	Volvulus	1
	Gastro-enteritis/colitis	3
Septicaemia (without meningitis)	Meningococcus	4
	Escherichia coli	2
	Waterhouse-Friderichsen (no organism isolated)	2
Accident/trauma (excluding head injury)	Hanging/wedging	5
	Choking	2
	Drowning	2
	Other	1
Metabolic	MCAD[1]	3
Other	Neonatal herpes simplex	1
	Ectodermal dysplasia	1
		n = 80

[1]MCAD = medium chain acyl Co-A dehydrogenase deficiency

Table 6.3 Ancillary tests indicating the major or probable contributory cause of death

	Major cause of death	Probable contributor to death	Total	%
Histology	49	5	54	67
Bacteriology	17	2	19	11
Virology	5	0	5	6.25
Frozen section	3	0	3	3.75
X-ray	2	1	3	3.75
Vitreous electrolytes	0	0	0	0

Table 6.4 Positive histology indicating the major or probable contributory cause of death by organ system

Organ system	Number of cases with positive histology
Respiratory tract	20
Central nervous system	16
Cardiovascular system	8
Gastro-intestinal	6
Endocrine (adrenal)	5
Genito-urinary	1
Skeletal	3

6.3.4   **A comparison of the causes of death given for SUDI by the confidential enquiry, local pathologists and regional paediatric pathologists**

Because of the anonymisation of records prior to the confidential enquiry process, it was not possible to make a direct comparison of the conclusions of the confidential enquiry with those of the regional pathology reviewers for individual cases. However, the high level of ascertainment for both the pathology and the case-control studies (97% and 98%, respectively) allow overall comparisons to be made between these two studies (Table 6.5).

The comparative study showed that:

• the final conclusions of the local case discussion meeting, the confidential enquiry panel, and the regional pathology coordinators review were in general agreement as to the broad grouping of causes of the deaths - at least as far as their classification into SIDS and non-SIDS is concerned.

• the major limitation of the assessment by the regional pathology coordinators was the lack of information concerning the circumstances of the death and family background, which were important factors for both the local case discussion meetings and the confidential enquiry in assessing whether deaths were accidental or non-accidental. This particularly applied to those deaths attributed by the confidential enquiry panels to probable or possible smothering by a parent.

• the initial assessments of the local pathologists (which would usually be incorporated into the registered causes of death) were substantially different from all other assessments. The local pathologists sometimes attributed deaths to causes, which were not considered as sufficient causes of death by an expert paediatric pathologist. However, this possible misclassification of deaths at the initial postmortem examination involved both an over-interpretation of relatively minor pathological changes and a failure to identify the significance of real pathology (e.g. fractures). The real level of discrepancy between the attributed causes of death between the local pathologists and the regional reviewers was thus greater than the overall figures would suggest. These findings are remarkably similar to those of the Knowelden study of post-neonatal deaths in the 1970s[4].

Table 6.5 A comparison of the causes of death given for sudden unexpected deaths in infancy by different groups in the CESDI study

Cause of death attributed by:	SIDS		Explained SUDI	
	n	%	n	%
Local pathologist	315	70	135	30
Regional pathology coordinator	369	82	80	18
Confidential enquiry or local case discussion	363	80	93	20

6.4   **CONCLUSION**

The single most useful component of the investigation of sudden unexpected death in infancy is a very detailed clinical history, which should include a detailed description of the precise circumstances of the death.   This will not only point to cases with a complete explanation for death prior to autopsy, but in some cases indicates the organ system that requires particularly careful investigation.

It is not always possible even for experienced pathologists to recognise pulmonary infection or fatty change in the liver from macroscopic appearances, or predict which cases will have positive cultures of blood or cerebrospinal fluid. This confirms the necessity of following a protocol in carrying out postmortem examinations of infants who have died suddenly and unexpectedly.

Histology was the single most useful ancillary investigation, and so is recommended in every case. Samples should be taken from the upper and lower respiratory tract, including all five lobes of the lungs. A frozen section of liver for fat is currently the most easily available screening test for MCAD, and should be undertaken in every case. Residual tissue should be saved as a source of DNA analysis in case the frozen section is positive.

Vitreous electrolytes did not demonstrate a single case of unsuspected dehydration or salt poisoning but did confirm the stability of sodium and urea values for several days after death, and that mild dehydration is a common association of systemic illness and a possible contributor to death.

Routine radiology demonstrated fractures in less than 2% of cases in which this was undertaken. In all of these cases, radiological examination was indicated by the history, or a fracture was found at postmortem examination, prompting skeletal survey. A concern was that in all but one case where there was also blunt injury to the head, death was attributed to natural causes. It is important that X-rays are reviewed by an experienced radiologist, and that any fractures are drawn to the attention of somebody experienced in child abuse.

There have been several developments in the field of unexpected infant death since the original CESDI SUDI postmortem protocol was devised.

The CESDI investigation itself has demonstrated the frequency of drug abuse among parents whose children die suddenly and unexpectedly. There is no European study demonstrating a significant incidence of poisoning by recreational or therapeutic drugs in babies who die suddenly and unexpectedly. Nevertheless, consideration should be given to toxicological analyses in individual cases, and appropriate samples should ideally be retained as a routine in case questions are raised later.

Recent work has suggested that the finding of abundant intra-alveolar haemosiderin in the lungs of babies who die suddenly and unexpectedly can be associated with episodes of previous imposed upper airway obstruction. Special examination for iron in the lung may be a useful screening test which may alert the pathologist in some cases, but does not exclude suffocation in others.

Measurement of the rectal temperature as soon as death is certified may support a clinical suspicion of overheating and help clarify the physiological mechanism of death when there is no finding at postmortem examination. However, there are no data available about the normal behaviour of body temperature after death in infants.

Sudden infant death syndrome is a diagnosis of exclusion. In this context, negative results are positive findings. SIDS is now less common than formerly, and so the proportion of explained natural and unnatural deaths among the cot death population has increased. In this study, 18% of deaths were fully explained by postmortem, and this is probably a minimum figure. The findings in cases in which a full range of ancillary tests was undertaken demonstrate the likelihood that causes of death were missed in those in which tests were not carried out. The percentage of positive results for each test in which the result was recorded is given in Table 6.6. These figures represent the maximum chance of missing a significant result if these tests are not carried out.

Table 6.6 Ancillary tests: percentage of significant positive results in those cases in which the result was recorded

Ancillary test	Positive results %
Histology	15.5 - 22
Blood culture (single organism plus/minus abnormal histology)	2.4 - 5
CSF[1] (single organism plus/minus abnormal histology)	2.5 - 6
NPA/lung virology	4.5
X-ray (healing fractures)	2
Frozen section of liver (MCAD[2] deficiency)	1

[1]CSF - cerebrospinal fluid
[2]MCAD - medium chain acyl Co-A dehydrogenase

The importance of full investigation and documentation, including negative findings, may only become apparent when a subsequent child dies, either of natural or unnatural causes. A suggested protocol based on the analysis of the ancillary investigations undertaken in these 450 cases, and their influence on the final diagnosis, is given below (Table 6.7).

Table 6.7 An evidence-based protocol for postmortem examination of sudden unexpected infant deaths

Full history	Birth history
	Medical history
	Social history
	Health and events preceding death
	Exact circumstances of death
Full autopsy	All body cavities
Full histology	Five lobes of lung, upper and lower respiratory tract
	All major organ systems
	Any lesion
Bacteriology	Blood
	Cerebrospinal fluid
	Lung
	Spleen swab
	Any lesion
Virology	Nasopharyngeal aspirate
	Lung
	Bowel contents (if indicated by history or postmortem findings)

Vitreous electrolytes	(Sodium and urea) Omit if eyes needed for histology (e.g. retinal haemorrhage)
Frozen section of liver for fat	All cases Save frozen liver
X-ray	Either all cases, or any cases in which history or postmortem suggests trauma
Consider	Rectal temperature Lung section stained by Perls' method Toxicology Skin, muscle, costochondral junction Fibroblast culture

REFERENCES

1. Department of Health. Additional guidelines for postmortem investigation associated with studies of sudden infant deaths: in The Confidential Enquiry into Stillbirths and Deaths in Infancy: First Report. London: DoH, 1993: appendix F, annex C.

2. Royal College of Pathologists. Guidelines for Postmortem Examinations after Sudden Unexpected Deaths in Infancy. London: RCP, 1993.

3. Gilbert, R, Rudd, P, Berry, PJ, Fleming, PJ, Hall, E et al. Combined effect of infection and heavy wrapping on the risk of sudden infant death, Archives of Diseases in Childhood, 1992; 67: 171- 7.

4. Knowelden, J, Keeling, J and Nicholl, JP. A Multicentre Study of Post-neonatal Mortality. University of Sheffield: Medical Care Research Unit, 1984.

ACKNOWLEDGEMENTS

Summarised by:
Dr Steve Gould, Consultant Pathologist, John Radcliffe Hospital, Oxford
Dr Jean Keeling, Consultant Pathologist, Royal Hospital for Sick Children, Edinburgh

From:
The pathology study: the contribution of ancillary pathology tests to the investigation of unexpected infant death. The CESDI SUDI Studies 1993-1996. London: The Stationery Office, 2000.

Authors:

Professor Jem Berry, Professor of Paediatric Pathology, St Michael's Hospital, Bristol.

Dr Eleanor Allibone, CESDI Pathologist, Yorkshire Region.

Dr Pat McKeever, Paediatric Pathologist, Leicester Royal Infirmary.

Dr Isabella Moore, Consultant Pathologist, Southampton General Hospital.

Dr Chris Wright, Consultant Paediatric Pathologist, Royal Victoria Hospital, Newcastle-upon-Tyne.

Professor Peter Fleming, Professor of Infant Health and Developmental Physiology, Royal Hospital for Sick Children, Bristol.

7

COMMUNICATIONS REVIEW

7.1   BACKGROUND

Successive CESDI Annual Reports have highlighted the apparent contribution of deficiencies in communication to sub-optimal care leading to stillbirth and infant death. These deficiencies include communication problems between professionals and parents, and poor communication between professionals, including inadequate record keeping. As CESDI was not set up to systematically investigate these issues, and as hospital records do not often record all communication problems, it is difficult to assess the extent of the impact of communication failure on deaths. In addition, as the information available to CESDI is based on clinical records, it does not include parental information about communication problems.

In response to these difficulties, the National Perinatal Epidemiology Unit (NPEU) was commissioned to undertake a review of the relevant research literature, as well as to undertake a small study of the experience of researchers who have included parent interviews in their work.

7.2   LIMITATIONS

The lack of denominator data makes it extremely difficult to draw any firm conclusions about the relationship between poor communication and adverse outcome. In addition, the number of papers that explicitly looked at poor communication as a factor in sub-optimal care is small, and therefore secondary evidence, based on inferring problems of communication in other types of suboptimal care was relied upon.

As a result it is difficult to estimate the extent of the problem of poor communication in perinatal and infant care, and to assess the link between poor communication and stillbirth and infant death. However, the studies looked at as part of the review provided some information about the types of communication problem that occur.

7.3   DOES POOR COMMUNICATION CONTRIBUTE TO STILLBIRTHS AND INFANT DEATHS?

7.3.1   Between professionals and parents

Between professionals and parents, there were two recurring themes, and the first of these related to the perceived failures of professionals to explain, inform or listen to mothers. Typically these occurred in the context of reduced fetal movements or other changes in pregnancy. Maternal delay in reporting reduced fetal movements, and inadequate response on the part of professionals to this and similar information from mothers, both antenatally and during labour, were the most common examples of this type of problem.

The second type, often referred to as "maternal non-compliance" occurred both antenatally; i.e. maternal failure to attend for antenatal care, or refusal to follow health care advice; and during labour, i.e. delay in seeking help or going to hospital, or refusal or delay in accepting interventions, usually in response to fetal distress.

These suggest communication problems around relationship building and information exchange, particularly in the antenatal period, although in the period immediately before labour and during labour similar issues arose.

7.3.2   **Between professionals**
Less information was available about communication failures between professionals. This may be because poor communication between professionals occurs less frequently. Alternatively it may be more difficult to identify poor inter-professional communication from available sources of information. Records of care form one way in which professionals communicate with one another, but not all communication between professionals is recorded. Furthermore, while the medical record may well contain information on the results of a breakdown of communication, it may not be clear from the record that poor communication was at the root of the problem, and other factors such as a lack of staff available may have had an impact.

However, the review identified three specific problem areas relating to inter-professional communication:

- During the antenatal period, problems were identified of continuity of care and information exchange between professionals, particularly with reference to the care of women at risk of various obstetric complications.
- Delays in responding to indications of fetal distress, often as a result of poor communication in the upward transfer of responsibility as a result of maternal or fetal distress.
- Poor record keeping, particularly during labour.

The studies reviewed provided little information on the mechanisms for these communication problems, although research into medical errors provides some support for the finding that communication problems occur when responsibility for care is being transferred. In particular a prospective study looking at the nature and causes of human errors in a six-bed medical-surgical intensive care unit in an Israeli teaching hospital, reported that the most common time for communication errors between nurses and doctors occurred shortly after doctors rounds, and at times of nurses' shift changes, suggesting problems with information exchange and transfer of responsibility.

Ong (1995)[1] identified three different purposes of communication, all of which are relevant to communication between professionals:

- Creating a good interpersonal relationship
- Exchanging information
- Making treatment-related decisions

It seems likely that different kinds of communication, with different purposes and requiring different skills, are needed at different stages of care. In addition the context for communication at different stages is likely to be very different. Whilst antenatal care usually takes place over a period of months with intermittent contact and often little urgency, intrapartum care takes place over a very short, more intensive time period, often with acute demands on those involved.

In contrast communication immediately before and during labour is likely to be focused on treatment-related decision-making and information exchange, but in the context of acute and emergent demands on those involved. It is worth noting that the issue of the context in which communication takes place is relevant to all communication, not just communication between professionals.

7.4   INTERVENTIONS TO IMPROVE COMMUNICATION AND THEIR EFFECTS ON PATIENT OUTCOME

7.4.1   Between patients and professionals

In maternity care, mother-held maternity records were effective in improving mother's perceptions of communication with their carers, involvement in their own care and control over their pregnancy. A small number of trials looking at the impact of training professionals in communication skills indicated an improvement in professional communication skills and this was reflected in patient satisfaction and knowledge, but the small number of trials preclude making any firm conclusions.

The number of trials of strategies to improve information exchange was very small. An earlier review identified specific areas in which the exchange of information between professionals and patients did not appear to be effective. Information relating to the significance of reduced or changed fetal movements appeared to be a particular problem and an area in which specific research could be of value. Evidence from a large randomised controlled trial has suggested that routine fetal movement counting alone is not effective in reducing the rate of stillbirths[2]. Women who were recommended to count fetal movements routinely every day during late pregnancy showed no reduction in antepartum death rates compared with control group women who were not instructed to monitor movements routinely. The authors suggested that compliance was an issue, and that improved compliance with counting, reporting and acting on reduced fetal movements might have improved performance, particularly in high risk cases. This suggests that further research into the effectiveness of strategies to improve the presentation of information relating to the significance of fetal movements might be of value.

All the trials examined were conduced in a sub-acute, general practice or outpatient setting, and therefore the usefulness of the findings, as a solution to intrapartum problems is questionable.

7.4.2 **Between professionals**

Good communication involves being given the information you need in a way you can understand, being listened to and being able to build relationships with caregivers. It may be that these themes apply as much to inter-professional communication as to communication between women and their carers, although there is less research in this area.

Only a small number of papers relating to inter-professional communication were identified, and the majority of these were descriptive or discussion papers, or poorly controlled studies. Therefore the most notable finding of this section of the review was the dearth of good quality research covering any aspect of communication between professionals. The trials that were identified all related to one aspect of communication, that between professionals in primary and secondary care. The results of two trials suggest that when general practitioners refer patients for consultant care they are likely to receive more feedback from consultants if they specifically ask for information.

The specific challenge for communication in maternity and perinatal care is that, because care is required for both mother and baby, a much wider group of health professionals may be involved than in many other areas of health care. The introduction of the National Maternity Record Project should go some way to solving problems of communication due to bad or inconsistent record design.

7.5 **THE ROLE OF PARENTAL INTERVIEWS**

This review considered the role of the parent interview in the research studies, as well as describing the views of a small number of people who have carried out interviews in the context of research with bereaved people.

In the early 1980's the NPEU reviewed the role of parental interviews; the recommendation made by the NPEU at the time was that parental interviews added information that could not be obtained elsewhere, and were acceptable to parents[3]. Other studies[4,5], also found that parents gave important information about poor care that was missing from the notes. In addition, Gilligan (1980)[5] found that the interviews were seen as helpful in raising staff awareness about care for bereaved parents.

More recent studies have found that, in addition to gathering data, contact with bereaved parents is likely to be helpful for most parents[6,7,8]. One limitation of information from parents is that it is collected retrospectively and events and recall bias may distort memories of care. However, support groups report that parents can talk about their memories of good aspects of care even in the most painful circumstances.

In the papers reviewed the timing of the interviews, and the professional conducting the interview, were determined by the needs of the studies therefore there is no clear evidence on what is best for parents.

Similarly there is no evidence available on whether one way of handling the collection of information for parents is likely to be better than another.

Interviewers often say that the completion of a short questionnaire is accompanied by a much longer informal discussion with parents.

When asked what effect this type of work had on them interviewers suggested that some sort of support should be built into the process so that they could talk to someone about difficult interviews. A study of health visitors in contact with families who had experienced a sudden infant death (in the course of their normal work) indicates that they felt distressed by the death and often turned to their own families for support[7].

REFERENCES
1.   Ong LML, de Haas JCJM, Hoos AM et al (1995). Doctor-patient communication: A review of the literature. Soc Sci Med; 40 (7): 903-18

2.   Grant AM, Elbourne DR, Valentin L, et al (1989). Routine formal fetal movement counting and risk of antepartum late death in normally-formed singletons. Lancet; ii (8659) : 345-9.

3.   Chalmers I (1984). Enquiry into perinatal death. A report on national perinatal surveillance prepared for the Department of Health and Social Security. Oxford: NPEU

4.   Brimblecombe FSW, Bastow M, Jones J, et al (1983). A suggested model for inquiries into perinatal and early childhood deaths in a health care district. Liverpool: Children's Research Fund.

5.   Gilligan M (1980b) The Midwife's contribution to counselling parents who have suffered a perinatal death. In : Research and the Midwife conference proceedings. London

6.   Rajan L and Oakley A. (1993). No pills for heartache: the importance of social support for women who suffer pregnancy loss. Journal of Reproductive and Infant Psychology; 11: 75-87

7.   Wright L. (1998) Sudden Infant death: How do health visitors cope? Community Practitioner; 71(3): 103-5

8. Kavanaugh K and Ayres L. (1998). "Not as bad as it could have been": assessing and mitigating harm during research interviews on sensitive topics. Re Nurs Health; 21 (1): 91-7

ACKNOWLEDGEMENTS

Summarised by:
Ms Helen Caddy, Project Manager, CESDI Secretariat
Mrs Sian Warriner, Midwife, CESDI Secretariat

from:
Communication Issues In Stillbirth And Infant Death:
A Review Of Communications within The CESDI Framework.
By Rachel Rowe, Jo Garcia, Alison Macfarlane and Leslie Davidson
National Perinatal Epidemiology Unit (NPEU). December 1999

8

CHANGING LOCAL PRACTICE

8. 1   **BACKGROUND**

The findings and recommendations of CESDI are important to both individuals and professional bodies. The messages are wide ranging and applicable to a broad spectrum of health workers, and at times, they are particularly relevant to parents. Findings and recommendations are disseminated to the professions via the Royal Colleges and statutory bodies, and increasingly, directly via Trusts and Health Authorities. Findings are distributed to the public through national and local media, voluntary organisations and support groups.

In addition, CESDI benefits from having a network of full-time Regional Co-ordinators and support staff, located across the fourteen former English Regions, and Wales and Northern Ireland. This unique network plays a significant role in the dissemination of the findings of CESDI. A study undertaken by the Office for Public Management in 1998 on the dissemination of CESDI findings to professionals found that awareness of CESDI is very high within those Trusts which have direct contact with Regional Co-ordinators. Direct involvement by local clinicians in CESDI activities such as data collection and attending panel enquiries enhances local awareness in hospitals. Regional Co-ordinators are responsible for specific populations, and they therefore get to know their units well, and are able to liaise effectively with local co-ordinators.

A key responsibility for Regional Co-ordinators is their involvement in the promotion of CESDI findings and recommendations to influence changes in practice within their particular Region. In recent Annual Reports the response to CESDI recommendations by national bodies such as the Royal Colleges and the UKCC have been included, but it was felt important also to highlight regional and local initiatives, and therefore this year's Changing Practice chapter provides some examples of initiatives undertaken at Regional and Unit level. It is worth noting however that awareness of CESDI influences care in less direct ways, for example in reinforcing current good practice, or in encouraging investment in training.

8. 2   **INCREASING LOCAL AWARENESS**

CESDI has recommended that protocols be put in place for the safe management of rare events such as shoulder dystocia, and the avoidance of ruptured uterus (5th Annual Report), and it is pleasing to note that many units have done so:

- In Wales local protocols for the management of shoulder dystocia, the use of syntocinon in the augmentation of labour, and the management of women in labour with a previous uterine scar have been introduced.
- Units in the South Western Region have introduced local protocols for shoulder dystocia and CTG monitoring.

- A number of protocols for managing particular situations have been developed in South East Thames (induction and augmentation in women with previous uterine scars, CTG interpretation, delivery of large babies, neonatal resuscitation).

CESDI has been instrumental in attaining improved quality services:

- Joint discussions between the CESDI teams in North East and North West Thames, and the two perinatal pathologists in the Region, identified a problem with a low uptake of postmortems in the Region and concerns were raised that too few postmortems were being carried out by the specialist pathologists. As a result, the joint team are looking at ways of including pathology in the regional specialist commissioning process. Discussions have now been expanded to include South East and South West Thames.
- One district in the Trent Region has purchased specialist paediatric pathology on the basis of the CESDI recommendations.

8. 3   **EMPHASISING THE IMPORTANCE OF RECORD KEEPING**
Record keeping has long been recognised as an essential part of the care given to a mother and her baby. Previous CESDI reports have drawn attention to deficiencies in record keeping, and the contribution of poor record keeping to sub-optimal care. Recommendations in the 3rd, 4th 5th and 6th Reports highlighted the need for "clear and adequate notes" and for "the quality of maternity records... to be improved".

It is encouraging that a number of initiatives have been implemented to improve record keeping:

- Local reviews and audits of record keeping have been undertaken (Anglia, North Western).
- The North Western Region collaborates with the local Supervising Authority for midwives concerning record keeping issues.
- Guidance for junior midwifery and medical staff on communications and record keeping e.g when to call for more senior assistance, has been developed in some units in South East Thames.
- A number of units in the Northern Region have redesigned their case notes and/or have introduced explicit guidelines concerning the dating and signing of written records.
- In Wales local annual training days on record keeping, with assistance from legal colleagues have been held.

8. 4   **IMPLEMENTING AND MONITORING PERFORMANCE**
Incorporating CESDI recommendations into contracts between Health Authorities and Trusts is a useful way of promoting the implementation of recommendations. The following incorporate CESDI recommendations into their contracts, although others may also do so:

- All Boards and Trusts in Northern Ireland.
- Portsmouth Health Authority in Wessex and The Channel Islands.
- West Kent Health Authority in the South East Thames Region.

In addition, most Regions regularly audit the uptake of CESDI recommendations, for example:

- In Yorkshire the Local Supervising Authority Responsible Midwifery Officer undertakes an annual audit of the implementation of all CESDI recommendations within all hospitals and health authorities in the Region.
- A telephone questionnaire was undertaken in the Trent Region by contacting all Heads of Midwifery to identify how CESDI recommendations had been implemented locally. A positive response was made in the majority of units with some or all recommendations being fulfilled or addressed.
- In the North Western Region a survey is about to commence which will evaluate the effectiveness of the dissemination process, and then consider the action taken by individual Trusts in response to the recommendations made in the last two reports.

8. 5 **CESDI'S ROLE IN CLINICAL GOVERNANCE AND RISK MANAGEMENT**
CESDI Regional Co-ordinators and their network of local contacts contribute regularly to perinatal mortality reviews, study days, workshops, conferences etc. at all levels, from small locally-based groups to regional and national conferences. CESDI's work is, by its nature, multidisciplinary and much is gained from pooling different professional perspectives. Direct feedback on the findings of individual panel enquiries is not currently permitted. However, much use is made of anonymised case notes in educational sessions and these are welcomed by unit staff.

- Many Regions undertake "Second Pass Panel" exercises, where the same cases are reviewed by local panels as well as by the regional panels.
- Workshops on shoulder dystocia and ruptured uterus are run in the Oxford Region, which also introduce clinical staff to the panel process and raises awareness of the importance of record keeping.
- The CESDI process and documentation is used in some Units in Wessex and The Channel Islands as a method of internal review, in addition to the regular perinatal mortality meetings.
- In one Unit in the North East Thames Region the CESDI process is used to look at "near misses", for example intrapartum asphyxia where the baby did not die.

Most CESDI Regions produce a Report relating to their own Region. These often include maternity and neonatal information relating to individual trusts which is often the only reliable source of local maternity statistics.

Regional meetings are held in which both local and national findings are presented, recommendations discussed and good practice shared. These meetings are popular mechanisms for cascading information to those on the "front line" as well as providing more localised feedback to those who have collected data and attended panel meetings.

In addition, CESDI can act as a setting for multidisciplinary regional consensus in related fields, for example a consensus meeting held in Mersey, comprising three representatives from each unit, resulted in the production of a standardised protocol for handling pre-eclampsia.

The role of CESDI in the development of local risk management schemes is also noted:

- The South Western Region has recently undertaken a survey of practice of obstetric units to identify amongst other issues the link between the CESDI findings and risk management.
- A postal questionnaire to assess risk management strategies has been undertaken throughout the Northern Region.

8. 6   ENCOURAGING CONTINUING EDUCATION AND TRAINING

Many of CESDI's recommendations have focused on specific aspects of education and training. The 4th Annual Report recommended that every hospital offering intrapartum care should have in place a regular rolling update/training programme in the use of CTGs for all professionals involved in intrapartum care. In addition, the 5th and 6th Annual Reports highlighted criticisms of CTG interpretation. Initiatives have been undertaken both at Regional level and locally in light of CESDI's findings.

Examples include:
- The West Midlands Region is currently focusing on training in intrapartum assessment, with a rolling workshop; "CTG Masterclass" starting with consultants, and including free installation of the "CTG Tutor" software in maternity units throughout the Region.
- CTG workshops, using CTGs from past CESDI cases, take place on a regular basis in the Mersey Region.
- In Trent, Nottingham City Hospital have developed guidelines for antenatal and intrapartum CTG interpretation, which have since been audited, and have now been implemented in two further hospitals.   (The Breech Focus Group (Chapter 3) used the guidelines in its audit of cases).

The 6th Annual Report highlighted that delivery suites should ensure that "the attending paediatrician has adequate experience in resuscitation skills". Examples of initiatives in this area include:
- A number of Units in the Anglia Region have introduced comprehensive neonatal resuscitation training for members of the paediatric team.
- In Northern Ireland a regional training programme in resuscitation for SHOs has been introduced and is held on a six-monthly basis.

- Units in South West Thames have funded staff to attend the Advanced Life Support in Obstetrics (ALSO) course.

8.7 COLLABORATION AND PARTNERSHIP

One of the key strengths of the Regional network is the flexibility each Regional office has in collaborating with other audit and research organisations.

- The North Western Perinatal Survey Unit (NWPSU) is currently working with the ORACLE Project on an audit and training programme for shoulder dystocia.
- The Northern Region collaborates with and assists the Regional Diabetic Pregnancy and Cerebral Palsy Registers.
- Mersey have undertaken an audit of the outcome of all livebirths born in the Region weighing less than 750g.
- South East Thames continue to support the Census on Neonatal Cot Usage.
- Regional audits of the quality of postmortem reporting are undertaken (North Western, Trent, Northern Ireland).
- Anglia have undertaken a survey of professional communication with women regarding fetal movements.
- South West Thames Region has collaborated for many years with the Regional Birth Survey, which collects data from every hospital in the Region and provides trend data. A similar survey is carried out in South East Thames.
- Many of the Regional Congenital Anomaly surveys work in conjunction with the CESDI network, and this ensures consistently high ascertainment which is fed back to the Office for National Statistics (ONS).

8. 8 PUBLICATIONS

A number of publications based on the work of CESDI have been produced by staff at Regional level. Articles have appeared in such diverse journals as the British Medical Journal, The Lancet, Midwives, Modern Midwife, The Diplomate, British Journal of Obstetrics and Gynaecology, and the Journal of Neonatal Nursing.

8. 9 CONTACT POINTS

CESDI Regional Co-ordinators are happy to provide further information on any of the initiatives described above. A list of names is found at the front of this Report, and their contact details are located on the website (www.cesdi.org.uk) or by contacting the CESDI Secretariat.

8. 10 FEEDBACK FROM READERS OF THE 6TH ANNUAL REPORT

For the past two years a reader questionnaire has been included with the Annual Report. Improvements arising from comments received from the 5th Report questionnaire include the introduction of a CESDI website on the World Wide Web, placing the current and some previous CESDI Reports onto the website, some style and layout alterations to the Report, and changes to the distribution of the Report.

Analysis of the questionnaires returned from the 6th Annual Report indicate the highest number of responses were from midwives (38% of total responses) and consultants (34%). More responses were received from senior professionals than from junior staff. The vast majority found the report and recommendations very or mostly useful. Nearly all respondents had read previous CESDI reports.

The educational value of CESDI's work was highlighted in a number of comments, in particular by midwives and midwifery lecturers. Typical comments included "An excellent aid to teaching student midwives" and "I include CESDI as a lecture topic on all midwifery refresher courses and post registration midwives' courses".

The use of anonymised case histories as examples was commented upon, and help to illustrate the issues.

One or two respondents commented on the presentation of some of the statistics and tables, and efforts have been made to simplify these. There were other suggestions regarding the availability of CESDI Reports, its layout and style, but in general, respondents felt that the Report was about right in terms of its size and length.

CESDI greatly appreciates the contributions made by the respondents to our questionnaire and we endeavour to implement their suggestions. We welcome any comments about this Report, either via the Questionnaire, the CESDI Website (www.cesdi.org.uk) or directly to the CESDI Secretariat at the address found on the back of the Report.

ACKNOWLEDGEMENTS

Author:
Ms Helen Caddy, CESDI Project Manager, CESDI Secretariat

With thanks to:
The Regional Co-ordinators who provided much of the information for this chapter.

9

CONCLUSIONS

The ability to provide accurate national clinical data in perinatal and infant medicine on the scale undertaken by CESDI is unique. This is especially important in rare circumstances such as intrapartum stillbirth and cot deaths. These have a major impact on parents and health professionals but occur so infrequently that lessons from individual events are limited. The multidisciplinary approach used by CESDI enables failures of care to be more readily understood.

This is the 7th Annual Report of CESDI. It has addressed a number of topics that are of major current concern and has set out recommendations to address the deficiencies it has identified in the following areas of care.

9.1 **BREECH PRESENTATION AT ONSET OF LABOUR**
The management of breech presentation is contentious. Despite a lack of supportive data there is increasing use of Caesarean section as the routine mode of delivery in the UK. This is in part due to the widely held belief that birth trauma is responsible for a substantial part of the excess risk.

CESDI undertook a review of the management of all babies in 1994-1995 who were normally formed, weighed over 1.5kg at birth, were breech at the onset of labour and died due to an intrapartum related event.

A fifth of all the babies were born at home, many of them already delivering by the time a health professional attended. The unexpected nature of these events emphasises the need for explicit plans of action for dealing with an undiagnosed breech at home.

The undiagnosed breech was the largest category and is the group most at risk. Most mothers were admitted in the early stages of labour but diagnosis was often not made until late in the first stage.

Examination of the intrapartum management of those delivering in hospital found that:

- the single and most avoidable factor was suboptimal care given in labour rather than the conduct of the delivery itself.

- where the cardiotocograph (CTG) was available for review: there was clinical evidence of hypoxia in all but one case prior to delivery and there were delays in staff response to fetal compromise in nearly three quarters of cases. These ranged from 30 minutes up to 10 hours.

- the registrar was the professional most likely to be involved in the labour and delivery. This group contains experienced doctors but it is also a training grade and less than a fifth of these labours had more senior involvement at any stage: consultants were only informed in half of these cases prior to delivery. Inexperience at the time of delivery exacerbated the risk to an already hypoxic baby in some cases.

Pathology review confirmed the clinical findings that hypoxia was the commonest cause of death. Trauma as a sole cause contributed to one case. Less than a quarter of the postmortems included a systematic and comprehensive examination of factors relevant to the death of a breech baby born vaginally.

The Report recommends that Units should ensure that all staff are skilled in fetal surveillance regardless of the presentation of the baby. The most experienced available practitioner needs to be involved and should be present at a vaginal breech delivery.

Although failure to diagnose a breech is not viewed as a direct failure of care, it highlights the need for increased efforts to identify presentation both antenatally and in labour.

Not all professionals will have the opportunity for hands-on experience of breech delivery. Alternative approaches involving structured simulated training are recommended.

The postmortem examination should be conducted by a perinatal pathologist or pathologist with a special interest in perinatal work as important details are easily missed.

9.2   **OBSTETRIC ANAESTHESIA - DELAYS AND COMPLICATIONS**
Anaesthetists are an integral part of the obstetric care team. Their presence allows early consultation on the management of life-threatening obstetric complications. CESDI welcomed the help of the Obstetric Anaesthetists' Association (OAA) in reviewing anaesthetic delays and serious complications involved in the 1994-1995 intrapartum deaths. The inclusion of problems associated with general anaesthesia is especially important because this is a significant cause of morbidity which is often under-emphasised when death is the main outcome of review.

The review highlighted several important issues, in particular:

- general anaesthesia may result in serious life threatening complications to the mother.

- anaphylaxis of the mother in response to a general anaesthetic can result in unnecessary delays in delivery. The Report emphasises the need for *immediate* delivery of the baby in these circumstances. Epinephrine is the drug of choice for severe anaphylaxis. All staff should be aware of resuscitation techniques and should maintain their skills.

Delays in the provision of an anaesthetic were equally divided between problems of getting personnel into place and those of administering adequate anaesthesia for an urgent delivery. It was often not possible to determine whether the delays were due to inadequate staffing or to the unpredictable clustering of emergencies.

- It is therefore important that Trusts should review their practice and implement the standards outlined for obstetric anaesthesia services.

Communicating and defining the degree of urgency of the need to deliver a baby is particularly problematic. Choice of anaesthesia in an urgent situation depends on the skills and experience of the anaesthetist.

- In several cases long delays were associated with top-ups of epidural analgesia; unless they are going to be rapidly effective they should not be used in urgent situations.

Documentation of the reasons for delays, particularly in the administration of anaesthesia was poor; this limited the accuracy of a retrospective audit. The decision-to-delivery interval of 30 minutes or less is a pragmatic rather than an 'evidence-based' standard. Indeed, its feasibility has been questioned, and the review concluded:

- benchmarking nationally of the decision-to-delivery interval is a priority.

- Trusts need to ensure good documentation of anaesthetic events including the times of the decision-to-deliver, when the patient reaches the operating theatre, when the anaesthetist is informed, and when the baby is delivered. Systematic recording and evaluation of delays incurred is essential before progress can be made locally.

9.3   CARDIOTOCOGRAPH EDUCATION SURVEY

One of the recurrent themes noted by CESDI is the problem surrounding the use and interpretation of cardiotocographs (CTGs). Although this technology is acknowledged to be of limited value in identifying fetal hypoxia, the presence of abnormalities should always initiate a response from the health professional. CESDI recommended (4th Annual Report, 1997) that Trusts should provide adequate training in this subject. In 1998 a CESDI survey found that:

- training was almost universally available. Ability to confirm attendance existed for most (88%) midwives but for only half of the medical staff. The difference may be due to the more rigorous supervisory structure for midwifery.

- of the midwives involved, those most likely to be conducting the deliveries (grades E and F) were the least likely to have received training.

- of the doctors involved, locums and staff grades were the least likely to have access to training.

This led to the recommendation that:

- Trusts should be able to confirm that **all** staff involved in intrapartum care have received CTG training within the preceding year.

The survey found that many midwives are self-funded for this form of education:

- Self funding is inappropriate for training in a skill that is widely used to assess the wellbeing of the baby.

The content of education is the same for both medical and midwifery personnel and multidisciplinary education is available in over three-quarters of all units. However, there are often conflicts between service needs and education. Protected time is generally available for Specialist Registrars but not for other levels of staff.

The survey did not address the effectiveness of training; work in this area is limited although increased core knowledge has been demonstrated when interactive computer packages are compared to conventional methods. Relatively little use is made of the former approach.

The area least likely to be addressed in training was the medico-legal aspects of documentation and storage of CTGs. Risk management policies need to include information on this point.

| 9.4 | **SUDDEN UNEXPECTED DEATHS IN INFANCY - PATHOLOGY** |

Sudden Infant Death Syndrome (SIDS) is a diagnosis of exclusion - negative results are a positive finding. It is therefore important that a thorough postmortem examination is undertaken.

The CESDI study included the largest review ever undertaken of pathology findings in sudden unexpected infant death. A second review of postmortem examination findings in 450 cases was undertaken by a regional pathology co-ordinator, without knowledge of the conclusion reached by the local pathologists.

The original pathologists identified 30% of cases as being 'explained', but the reviewers confirmed this in only 18%. This was due to over-interpretation of relatively minor pathological changes and a failure to identify the significance of real pathology (eg fractures).

Use of tests varied with the type of pathologist: general, paediatric or forensic. The review concluded that a detailed clinical history, including the precise circumstances of the death, is the single most useful component of the investigation of sudden unexpected deaths in infancy and that histology is the single most useful ancillary investigation.

- histology should be performed in every case. Adequate histology was taken in 53% of cases investigated by general pathologists, 69% of cases seen by paediatric pathologists and 47% seen by forensic pathologists.

- the review highlights the need for a thorough postmortem examination; a recommended protocol is given in Chapter 6.

9.5   **COMMUNICATIONS**
Failures of communication are difficult to define and to measure. The term often encompasses a multitude of complex problems. The importance of this area in perinatal and infant death was the topic of a formal review and this is summarised in Chapter 7. The findings emphasise the dearth of good quality research on interventions designed to improve communication. Between professionals and parents there were two recurring themes:

- perceived failures of professionals to explain, inform or listen to mothers - typically in the context of reduced fetal movements.
- what is often referred to as 'maternal non-compliance'- failure to attend antenatal care or refusal to follow advice, suggesting problems around relationship building and information exchange.

9.6   **CHANGING LOCAL PRACTICE**
Learning from the lessons found at enquiries is essential to their purpose. This year CESDI has outlined some of the initiatives that are occurring at local level.

The Regional Co-ordinators have a valuable role in promoting changes in local practice. Examples are given in Chapter 8 but there is an emphasis on:

- collaboration between Trusts and between disciplines. For example consensus meetings to produce standardised protocols for a Region, introducing an enquiry process into review of diabetic pregnancies involving physicians and specialist nurses in this field.
- education and training - particularly skills based in CTG interpretation, neonatal resuscitation and obstetric emergencies.
- promoting internal review processes - local assessment of deaths and near misses using the enquiry process; standards of record keeping.
- introducing protocols within Trusts and standards into commissioning processes.

9.7   **CONCLUSION**

This 7th Annual Report has described and quantified deficiencies in the management of pregnant women and infants. Many are recurrent themes: problems with use and interpretation of CTGs; lack of senior involvement in high risk obstetrics; poor documentation in all disciplines; limited pathology services; and communication problems especially at times of urgency. Safety is fundamental to good practice and recognising where unnecessary risks occur in the service is part of the clinical governance remit.

Correcting some of these deficiencies is under the control of local providers. But what local initiatives cannot do is to provide national overviews, standards, and benchmarking information. The absence of the latter often precludes rational assessment. The '30 minute' decision-to-delivery interval is a good example: is this a practical standard with current facilities? How can this be judged until data from all Trusts is available? CESDI has confirmed that delays in anaesthesia resulted in the death of some babies. Did this occur by chance or was it due to inadequate provision of services? Unless reliable information is available regarding staffing levels and quality of services, improvements will be limited. CESDI is uniquely placed through its Regional network to gather such information. This will facilitate the clinical governance process and help to improve the standards of care for mothers and babies.

ACKNOWLEDGEMENTS

Particular thanks are due to the considerable contribution of the district co-ordinators and the many others based throughout England, Wales and Northern Ireland, who often without recognition and in their own time, undertake work for CESDI.

Author:
Dr Mary Macintosh, Director, CESDI

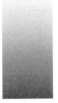

APPENDIX 1 - CESDI WORKING GROUPS

MEMBERS OF THE COMMUNICATIONS WORKING GROUP

Lady Shirley Littler (Chair)
Chair of the National Advisory Body

Dr Patrick Cartlidge
Consultant Neonatal Paediatrician
University of Wales College of Medicine

Mrs Eileen Hutton, OBE
Parental Voice

Mrs Linda Lamont
Parental Voice

Dr Mary Macintosh
CESDI - Director

Professor Andrew Wilkinson
Professor of Paediatrics
University of Oxford

Dr Gavin Young
General Practitioner
Temple Sowerby, Cumbria

MEMBERS OF THE RAPID REPORT FORM WORKING GROUP

Dr Mary Macintosh (Chair)
Director
CESDI Secretariat

Professor Eva Alberman
Professor of Epidemiology
St Bartholomews, London

Dr Patrick Cartlidge
Consultant Neonatal Paediatrician
University of Wales College of Medicine

Professor Geoffrey Chamberlain
Emeritus Professor,
Singleton Hospital, Swansea

Dr Jean Chapple
Consultant Perinatal Epidemiologist
Kensington, Chelsea and Westminster
Health Authority

Ms Grace Edwards
CESDI - Regional Co-ordinator

Dr Steve Gould
Consultant Paediatric Pathologist
John Radcliffe Hospital, Oxford

Ms Juliette Greenwood
Critical Care Services Manager
The Hospital for Sick Children, London

Dr Patricia Hamilton
Consultant in Neonatal Paediatrics
St George's Hospital, London

Mr Steven Bailey
CESDI -Data Analyst

Ms Alison Macfarlane
Reader in Perinatal and Public Health
Statistics
National Perinatal Epidemiological Unit,
Oxford

Ms Stephanie Roberts
CESDI - Regional Co-ordinator

Mr Jim Thornton
Reader in Obstetrics and Gynaecology
University of Leeds

MEMBERS OF THE CLASSIFICATION WORKING GROUP

Dr Steve Gould (Chair)
Consultant Paediatric Pathologist
John Radcliffe Hospital, Oxford

Professor Eva Alberman
Professor of Epidemiology
St Bartholomew's Hospital, London

Mrs Beverley Botting
Statistician
Office for National Statistics

Dr Patrick Cartlidge
Consultant Neonatal Paediatrician
University of Wales College of Medicine

Ms Nirupa Dattani
Senior Research Officer
Office for National Statistics

Ms Grace Edwards
CESDI - Regional Co-ordinator

Mr Charles Lee
CESDI - IT Specialist

Dr Mary Macintosh
CESDI - Director

Dr Sheila Macphail
Senior Lecturer in Obstetrics
University of Newcastle

Dr Gillian Penney
Programme Co-ordinator
Scottish Programme for Clinical Effectiveness in
Reproductive Health

Ms Stephanie Roberts
CESDI - Regional Co-ordinator

Dr Maureen Scott
CESDI - Regional Co-ordinator

Dr Chris Wright
Consultant Paediatric Pathologist
Royal Victoria Infirmary, Newcastle Upon Tyne

APPENDIX 2 - RAPID REPORT FORM 1998

CESDI (Confidential Enquiry into Stillbirths and Deaths in Infancy)

Survey Number

Notification Form - 1998

1. How was this case defined? Note:- It is possible for a case to be both a registrable death (stillbirth or neonatal death) AND a legal abortion

Late fetal loss (20+0-23+6 weeks) 1	Stillbirth (24+weeks) 2	Early Neonatal Death (age 0 - 6 days) 3	Late Neonatal Death (age 7 - 27 days) 4	Post Neonatal Death (28 to 364 days) 5

2. Legal Abortion? (Under 1967/92 Abortion Act) YES 1

MOTHER

3. Mother's surname

4. First name   5. Hospital No.

6. Mother's usual residential address at time of delivery/birth

7. Postcode

8. Mother's date of birth _____ Day _____ Month _____ Year   or _____ or _____ N.K.   tick if Estimated age 9

9. Ethnic group of mother: White 1, Black African 2, Black Carib. 3, Black other 4, Indian 5, Pakistani 6, Bangladeshi 7, Chinese 8, N.K. 9, OTHER (specify) 0

10 Parity — No. of previous pregnancies of 24+ weeks ONLY   tick if Not Known 9

THIS PREGNANCY

11. What was first day of the Last Menstrual Period (LMP)   Day Month Year   N.K. 9

12. What was the agreed working Estimated Date of Delivery (EDD) just before birth?   Day Month Year

13. Gestation at Birth (best estimate) _____ weeks + _____ days

14. Date and Time of delivery / birth   Day Month Year   24 hr clock

15. Intended place of delivery at booking — Name of Unit / Place

16. Actual place of delivery — Name of Unit / Place

17. Reason for change between planned and actual place of delivery
- No change 1
- Change of address during pregnancy 2
- Clinical reasons before labour 3
- Other reasons before labour 4
- Clinical reasons after onset of labour 5
- Other reasons after onset of labour 6
- Unintentionally after onset of labour 7
- Not known 9

18. Number of fetuses / babies this pregnancy — All identifiable fetuses at delivery, including papyraceous   tick if Not Known 9

19. Birth Order This Fetus / Baby (0, 1, 2, 3 etc) — 0 = Singleton   tick if Not Known 9

20. Maternal Insulin or Impaired Glucose Tolerance this pregnancy — Was there any history of maternal diabetes or glucose intolerance in this pregnancy? Yes 1 No 2   If YES b. Was this diagnosed during this pregnancy? YES 1 No 2   c. Was this Insulin treated? YES 1 No 2

21. Presentation just prior to delivery   Cephalic 1 Breech 2 Other 3   Tick here if N.K. 9

22. Mode of Delivery   Spont. Vaginal 1 Low Forceps 2 N.K. 9 Other forceps (inc. Kiellands) 3 Ventouse 4 Assisted Manual 5 Emergency Caesn. Sec. 6 Planned C.S. 7 Other 8

Please give name or whom to contact for further information:

position / post:

contact address:

Telephone number:

BABY / INFANT

23. Baby's surname

24. First name   25. Hospital No.

26. Baby's residential address at time of death if different from Q6.

27. Postcode

Region of Residence — CESDI regional office to complete

28. Sex of fetus/baby   MALE 1   FEMALE 2   Indeterminate 3   N.K. 9

29. Birth Weight (kg) (Earliest possible please)   Tick if □ N.K. □ Never recorded 0

30. Place of death (LIVEBIRTHS ONLY) — Name of Unit / Place

31. Date and Time death was FIRST diagnosed (confirmed) — Live births only   Day Month Year   24 hr clock   tick if time estimated

32. Timing of death — Stillbirths and Late Fetal Losses ONLY
- before admission, not in labour 1
- before admission, probably in labour 2
- after admission but before labour 3
- after admission, during labour 4
- N.K. 9

33. Signs/observations at birth - tick all features observed in the first hour after delivery   if N.K. 9
- Audible cry 1
- Spontaneous breathing 2
- effort or active body movts.
- Spontaneous heart beat 3
- No maceration - no signs of life 4
- Early maceration 5
- Advanced maceration 6

34. Discharge Home after birth or neonatal care — Live births ONLY — Was baby ever discharged home after birth? YES 1 No 2 N/K 9   If YES, date and time of readmission to hospital   Day Month Year   24 hr clock

35. CAUSE OF DEATH - CLINICAL DETAILS   for office use

a. Main diseases or conditions in fetus / infant

b. Other diseases or conditions in fetus / infant

c. Main maternal diseases or conditions affecting fetus/neonate

d. Other maternal diseases or conditions affecting fetus/neonate

e. Other relevant causes or comments

36. EXTENDED WIGGLESWORTH CLASSIFICATION (see guidelines) — Text   enter number

37. FETAL AND INFANT CLASSIFICATION (see guidelines) — Text   enter number

38. OBSTETRIC CLASSIFICATION (see guidelines) — Text   enter number

39. POST MORTEM (AUTOPSY)
- Held/being arranged 1
- Not requested 2
- Requested but consent not given 3   office use
- Coroners PM 4
- Parental consent but autopsy not done 5
- N/K

40. Date CESDI form completed   Day Month Year

95

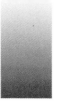

APPENDIX 3 - EXTENDED WIGGLESWORTH CLASSIFICATION

Category 1 **Congenital defect/malformation (lethal or severe):** Only **lethal** or potentially lethal congenital malformation should be included here. **Serious biochemical abnormalities** such as **Tay Sach's disease** and any known single gene defects known to have a high risk of death should be included.

Category 2 **Unexplained antepartum fetal death:** Most late fetal losses should be coded here. Where a live born baby dies due to problems during the antepartum period, code this as 'other specific causes'.

Category 3 **Death from intrapartum 'asphyxia', 'anoxia' or 'trauma':** This category covers any baby who would have survived but for some catastrophe occurring during labour. These babies will tend to be normally formed, stillborn or with poor Apgar scores, possible meconium aspiration or evidence of acidosis. Very premature infants (those less than 24 weeks gestation) may be asphyxiated at birth, but should not be entered in this category as a rule.

Category 4 **Immaturity:** This applies to live births only, who subsequently die from structural pulmonary immaturity, surfactant deficiency, intra ventricular haemorrhage, or their late consequences - including chronic lung damage.

Category 5 **Infection:** This applies where there is clear microbiological evidence of infection that could have caused death, e.g. maternal infection with Group B streptococci, rubella, parvovirus, syphilis etc; or in the case of a baby dying with overwhelming sepsis.

Category 6 **Due to other specific causes:** Use this if there is a specific recognisable fetal, neonatal or paediatric condition not covered under the earlier categories. Examples include:

1) *fetal* conditions; twin-to-twin transfusion and hydrops fetalis;

2) *neonatal* conditions; pulmonary haemorrhage, pulmonary hypoplasia due to prolonged loss of liquor (primary hypoplasia being classed as a malformation), persistent transitional circulation (in the absence of infection, aspiration or surfactant deficiency), blood loss unassociated with trauma (e.g. vasa praevia);

3) *paediatric* conditions; malignancy and acute abdominal catastrophe (such as volvulus without antecedent congenital malrotation).

Category 7 **Due to accident or non-intrapartum trauma:** Confirmed non-accidental injury should be coded here. If only suspected, code as a sudden unexpected death cause unknown (category 8)

Category 8 **Sudden infant death, cause unknown:** This will include all infants in whom the cause is unknown or unsuspected at the time of death. Modification due to post mortem information should be notified later.

Category 9 **Unclassifiable:** To be used as a last resort. Details must be given if this option is ticked.

DEFINITION OF THE TERMS USED IN THE OBSTETRIC (Aberdeen) CLASSIFICATION

CONGENITAL ANOMALY. Any genetic or structural defect arising at conception or during embryogenesis incompatible with life or potentially treatable but causing death.

ISOIMMUNISATION. Death ascribable to blood group incompatibility, rhesus (3) or non rhesus (4).

PRE-ECLAMPSIA. Diastolic blood pressure of 90 mmHg or more on two separate days after 20 weeks gestation (140 days) with significant proteinuria in the absence of existing hypertensive disease prior to pregnancy. Without APH (5) or with APH (6).

ANTEPARTUM HAEMORRHAGE (APH), after 20 weeks gestation (140 days) whether revealed or not, excluding antepartum haemorrhage secondary to pre-eclampsia (which is classified under pre-eclampsia). Minor degrees of haemorrhage at the start of labour (a show), and haemorrhage due to a cervical erosion or polyp should be ignored, but significant or recurrent bleeding of uncertain origin that is fairly closely followed by preterm labour should not be ignored.

MECHANICAL. Any death from uterine rupture and those deaths from birth trauma, or intrapartum asphyxia that are associated with problems in labour such as disproportion, malpresentation, cord prolapse, cord compression, or breech delivery in babies of 1000g or more. If there is no evidence of difficulty in labour, deaths from asphyxia or trauma should be classified as unexplained.
Antepartum deaths associated with cord entanglement in the absence of strong circumstantial evidence that cord compression caused death (eg, fetal death soon after external version) should also be classified as unexplained.

MATERNAL DISORDER. Include maternal trauma (such as a road traffic accident), diabetes, appendicitis, and cardiac disease etc, if severe enough to jeopardise the baby. Include significant renal disease or essential hypertension known to be present before pregnancy. Also include symptomatic and asymptomatic maternal infection when this resulted in the death of the baby.

MISCELLANEOUS. Specific fetal and neonatal conditions only. Do not include conditions directly ascribable to prematurity or anoxia before birth, because these deaths are attributable to the relevant underlying obstetric disorder or are unexplained (see below). Include, however, specific fetal conditions (eg, twin-to-twin transfusion) or neonatal conditions (eg, inhalation of milk) where these are not directly ascribable to intrapartum anoxia or preterm delivery. Include, also postnatally acquired infection, except in babies of less than 1000g; here the reason for the ventilator dependancy or low birthweight is the codeable factor.

UNEXPLAINED. Deaths with no obstetric explanation, including unexplained antepartum stillbirths, deaths resulting from unexplained preterm delivery (including hyaline membrane disease, intraventricular haemorrhage, etc) and cases of intrapartum anoxia or trauma if the baby weighed less than 1000g at birth or delivery without any obvious associated mechanical problem. Cases should be subclassified into those babies weighing 2500g or more (20) and those of less than 2500g (21) at birth.

UNCLASSIFIABLE. Cases where little or nothing is known about pregnancy or delivery and that cannot be fitted into any of the above categories. Use this category as sparingly as possible.

OBSTETRIC (Aberdeen) CLASSIFICATION

Categories at the head of the list take priority over those lower down. Only ONE answer applies — **it is the lowest numbered category that adequately describes the death.**

Code	Category
	Congenital anomaly:— any structural or genetic defect incompatible with life or potentially treatable but causing death.
1	Neural tube defects
2	Other anomalies
	Isoimmunisation:— death ascribable to blood group incompatibility
3	Due to Rhesus (D) antigen
4	Due to other antigens
	Pre-eclampsia
5	Without APH
6	Complicated by APH
	Antepartum Haemorrhage (APH)
7	With placenta praevia
8	With placental abruption
9	APH of uncertain origin
	Mechanical
10	Cord prolapse or compression with vertex or face presentation
11	Other vertex or face presentation
12	Breech presentation
13	Oblique or compound presentation, uterine rupture etc.
	Maternal disorder
14	Maternal hypertensive disease
15	Other maternal disease
16	Maternal infection
	Miscellaneous
17	Neonatal infection
18	Other neonatal disease
19	Specific fetal conditions
	Unexplained
20	Equal or greater than 2.5kg
21	Less than 2.5kg
22	Unclassifiable

DEFINITION OF THE TERMS USED WHEN CLASSIFYING THE MAIN FETAL AND NEONATAL FACTORS INVOLVED IN PERINATAL DEATH.

CONGENITAL ANOMALY. Any genetic or structural defect arising at conception or during embryogenesis incompatible with life or protentially treatable but causing death. Separate out deaths associated with a neural tube defect and death caused by chromosomal, cardiac or renal abnormality from deaths due to other miscellaneous or multiple abnormalities.

ISOIMMUNISATION. Death ascribable to blood group incompatibility.

ASPHYXIA BEFORE BIRTH (whether the baby is stillborn or not). Specify whether the insult originated before (8) or during (9) labour. All non-malformed stillborn babies are arbitrarily classified as dying of asphyxia unless death is due to a specific recognisable condition such as idiopathic hydrops fetalis, twin-to-twin transfusion etc, or there is evidence of malformation, isoimmunisation, trauma or infection. It would be assumed that asphyxia developed during labour unless there is reasonable evidence to the contrary if the baby was alive when labour started.

BIRTH TRAUMA. Death during or after birth due to rupture of the liver, splenic avulsion, fracture/dislocation of the occipital bone, or due to serious damage of the falx, tentorium, great cerebral vein or cervical spine during delivery. Where there is clinical or postmortem evidence of both asphyxia and trauma, death should be ascribed to asphyxia before birth (see above) unless it is clear that trauma is the more important factor.

SEVERE PULMONARY IMMATURITY. Babies with structural immaturity of the lung so gross as to render sustained ventilatory support unsatisfactory from the outset. Such babies are almost always less than 27 weeks gestation at birth.

HYALINE MEMBRANE DISEASE (HMD). Death due to pulmonary immaturity or surfactant deficiency or its late consequences. Specify whether there was significant periventricular bleeding (or infarction) (13) or secondary infection (14) as well.

INTRACRANIAL HAEMORRHAGE (or infarction). Exclude intraventricular and periventricular haemorrhage associated with potentially lethal HMD (12-14), and other haemorrhage secondary to trauma (10) or asphyxia before delivery (8 or 9). Separate deaths due to intraventricular or periventricular haemorrhage or infarction (15) including periventricular leukomalacia (conditions that are normally associated with preterm delivery) from other intracerebral haemorrhages (such as subarachnoid or cortical haemorrhage) or cerebrovascular occlusion of the type more normally seen in babies born at term (16).

INFECTION (including necrotising enterocolitis). Include antepartum as well as postpartum infection but exclude infection secondary to treatment for HMD. Separate deaths from necrotising enterocolitis from other deaths, and indicate, in the remaining cases, whether the infection was thought to have been acquired before the onset of labour, during delivery, or after birth. Specify site and organism.

MISCELLANEOUS. Death due to other specific fetal and neonatal conditions. Specific fetal conditions include tumours, isoimmunisation, unexplained hydrops fetalis and death due to the twin-to-twin transfusion syndrome. Specific neonatal conditions include aspiration of milk or gastric contents, unexplained pulmonary haemorrhage, pulmonary hypoplasia due to prolonged loss of liquor (primary hypoplasia being classed as a malformation), persistent transitional circulation (in the absence of underlying aspiration or surfactant deficiency), and blood loss unassociated with trauma.

UNCLASSIFIABLE OR UNKNOWN. Other inadequately documented deaths, unattended deliveries, unexpected and unexplained cot deaths (22) unattended deliveries not otherwise classifiable (23) and other undocumented death (24)

FETAL AND NEONATAL FACTOR CLASSIFICATION

Categories at the head of the list take priority over those lower down. **Only one number can be applied to any one death.**

Code	Category
	Congenital anomaly:— any structural or genetic defect incompatible with life or potentially treatable but causing death.
1	Chromosomal defect
2	Inborn error of metabolism
3	Neural tube defect
4	Congenital heart defect
5	Renal abnormality
6	Other malformation
7	Isoimmunisation
	Asphyxia before birth
8	Antepartum asphyxia
9	Intrapartum asphyxia
10	Birth trauma
11	Severe pulmonary immaturity
	Hyaline Membrane Disease (HMD)
12	Hyaline Membrane Disease
13	HMD with IVH
14	HMD with infection
	Intracranial Haemorrhage (+Infarction)
15	Intraventricular haemorrhage (IVH)
16	Other intracranial bleeding
	Infection
17	Necrotising enterocolitis
18	Antepartum infection
19	Intrapartum infection
20	Post partum infection
21	Miscellaneous
	Unclassifiable or unknown
22	Cot death
23	Unattended delivery
24	Other undocumented death

APPENDIX 4 - INTRAPARTUM FETAL MONITORING GUIDELINES

Nottingham City Hospital (NHS Trust) Maternity Unit
Review October 2001. Version 2:1

INTRAPARTUM FETAL MONITORING FIRST STAGE

INTRAPARTUM CARDIOTOCOGRAPHS (CTG) are carried out when the mother is in labour. It is usual practice in this Unit to carry out a CTG on admission. If an admission CTG is not carried out e.g. the mother is in very advanced labour or she declines to be monitored, this should be documented on the partogram. CTGs should be carried out for a minimum of 20 minutes and classified as **NORMAL**, **SUSPICIOUS** or **PATHOLOGICAL** and documented on the partogram.

- **CTGs must always be interpreted in the light of the clinical evidence and each individual situation.** Clinical guidelines are guidelines only. The interpretation and application of clinical guidelines will remain the responsibility of the individual clinician. If in doubt, contact a senior colleague. Caution is advised when using guidelines after the review date (Nottingham City Hospital, 1999).

- It is possible that in some instances "doubling" of the fetal heart rate (FHR) may occur. It is also possible, though unlikely, to produce a CTG when there is no fetal heart rate. It is good practice to check in all cases that the FHR agrees with the electronic fetal monitoring (EFM) by Pinard stethoscope and by checking the mother's pulse rate. The mother's pulse rate and auscultated FHR should be written on the CTG at the beginning. CTG displays should be treated suspiciously if difficulty in adequately establishing FHR occurs (M.D.A. 1998). Check clock records correct time.

- Mothers with meconium-stained liquor, any other high risk factors or an epidural should be monitored continuously in labour. During siting of epidural where continuous CTG is indicated, FH should be intermittently monitored at 15 minute intervals and recorded on the monitor paper which should be kept running. EFM must be commenced following siting of epidural. In problem-free pregnancies administration of pethidine is not an indication for continuous EFM.

- Mothers with multiple pregnancies should be monitored continuously throughout labour. If the membranes are ruptured, it is possible to monitor one baby internally and the other baby externally. Twins should not be monitored externally using two machines. Mothers with intact membranes should have their babies electronically monitored consecutively with intermittent auscultation using the Doppler for the other twin, unless a CTG machine capable of carrying out two external CTGs is available.

- Cord blood gases should always be obtained when fetal blood sampling (FBS) has been performed in labour, or when delivery is expedited for abnormal CTG. Obtaining blood for cord gases is the responsibility of the person who delivers the baby.

INTRAPARTUM CTG DEFINITIONS

BASELINE RATE: The average level of the FHR when it is stable.
BASELINE VARIABILITY: The amount in beats per minute (bpm) by which the baseline varies.
ACCELERATION: Transient increase in the FHR of 15 bpm of 15 seconds or more.
DECELERATION: Slowing of the FHR below the baseline rate of 15 bpm or more for a period of 15 seconds or more.

TYPES OF DECELERATIONS

EARLY DECELERATION: deceleration which occurs with a regular pattern of uniform appearance with the low point coincident with the high point of the contraction (Gibb & Arulkumaran, 1992 p19).
VARIABLE DECELERATION: deceleration where the appearance and/or timing is variable (Gibb & Arulkumaran, 1992 p30).
LATE DECELERATION: recurrent uniform deceleration where the onset, nadir (lowest point) and recovery are out of phase with the contraction (Gibb & Arulkumaran, 1993 p19; Ingemarrson et al, 1993 p133).
PROLONGED DECELERATION: deceleration of < 100 bpm for 3 minutes or < 80 bpm for 2 minutes (Ingemarrson et al, 1993 p 193).

INTRAPARTUM CTG CLASSIFICATIONS

NORMAL CTGs will fulfil the criteria below in all 4 categories.
SUSPICIOUS CTGs are those which fall into 1 or more of the "suspicious" categories.
PATHOLOGICAL CTGs are those which fall into 1 or more of the "pathological" categories

CLASSIFICATION	BASELINE RATE (bpm)	VARIABILITY (bpm)	DECELERATIONS	ACCELERATIONS
NORMAL	110-150	10-25	None	Presence of accelerations is reassuring. Not enough evidence to comment on their absence in an otherwise normal CTG
SUSPICIOUS	100-109 151-170	5-9 or >25	Early deceleration Variable deceleration Single prolonged deceleration of up to 3 min	None
PATHOLOGICAL	<100 >170	< 5 for > 20 min	Late deceleration Prolonged deceleration of > 3 min	N/A
PATHOLOGICAL	"Sinusoidal" trace: smooth wave form of 2-5 cycles/min lasting > 20 min	None	N/A	N/A

ASSESSMENT & ACTION

- If the CTG is **NORMAL**, and the mother has a problem free pregnancy, the CTG should be discontinued and intermittent monitoring carried out. Intermittent monitoring is carried out every 15-30 minutes depending on the stage of labour by Pinard's stethoscope or Sonicaid. Mothers with a problem pregnancy should be monitored continuously.

- If the CTG is **SUSPICIOUS**, the CTG should be continued for a further 20 minutes and the **following possible causes considered and appropriate action taken**. If the CTG becomes normal during the next 20 minutes, it may be discontinued and intermittent monitoring carried out. If the CTG remains suspicious, referral should then be promptly made to an experienced SHO or Registrar who must carry out a complete review of the case. Consideration must be given to ascertaining directly fetal well being by doing FBS. If this is not possible, then immediate delivery must be considered.

POSSIBLE CAUSE	CONSIDER	ACTION
Inadequate quality of CTG	* Poor contact from external transducer, Fetal Scalp Electrode (FSE) not working or has become detached	* Check position of transducer / FSE * Consider applying FSE
Maternal Posture	* The mother's position	* Ensure mother is not lying flat
	* Is the mother hypotensive?	* Change position, record BP, give 500 ml IV fluids if appropriate
	* Has the mother just had a vaginal examination (VE)?	* Change position if appropriate
	* Has the mother just used a bedpan?	* Change position if appropriate
	* Has the mother been vomiting or had a vasovagal episode?	* Change position, give 500 ml IV fluids if appropriate
	* Has the mother just had an epidural sited or topped-up?	* Change position, give 500 ml IV fluids if appropriate
Maternal Tachycardia/ Pyrexia	* Is the mother anxious?	* Reassurance
	* Maternal infection?	* If temperature ≥ 37.8°C inform doctor & refer to Labour Suite guidelines
	* Tocolytic infusion?	* If pulse > 140 bpm, reduce rate and inform Doctor.
Drugs	* Opiates (injection or epidural)	* Expect CTG to return to normal in an hour
	* Tocolytic infusion	* If pulse > 140 bpm, reduce rate, inform doctor
Transitional Stage of Labour	* Is the cervix fully dilated?	* Carry out V.E. if presenting part not visible
Uterine Hyperstimulation Secondary Uterine Inertia	* Is the uterus over contracting?	* Stop syntocinon. If not on syntocinon, refer to doctor. Consider giving 500 mcg ritodrine
	* Consider uterine rupture/scar dehiscence	* Refer to doctor
Compromised Fetus Eg. IUGR, APH	* Is there meconium stained liquor or heavy bleeding?	* Inform doctor

- As soon as a CTG is recognised as **PATHOLOGICAL**, referral **must** be made immediately to an experienced SHO, Registrar or Consultant and the Labour Suite Co-ordinator, as fetal blood sampling (FBS) or delivery may be necessary. This should be done **prior** to administration of pethidine, epidural or initiation of syntocinon. Entonox may be given. The Labour Suite Co-ordinator may refer directly to the Consultant on call in the event of suspected mismanagement. The "decision to deliver" to delivery time interval should be as short as possible, ideally within 30 minutes.

DOCUMENTATION AND STORAGE

- All CTGs must be identified at the beginning of the trace by the mother's name and hospital number and dated. The fetal monitor's clock should be checked for accuracy and rechecked periodically. Events such as VE, drugs, use of bedpan etc. should be noted on CTG with the time.

- All CTGs should be signed by the midwife on completion and any action taken documented on the CTG. Any staff asked to review the CTG must sign it at the time of review. Time and mode of delivery should be recorded at the end of the CTG and signed by the midwife.

- For legal reasons and to fulfil UKCC rule 40 (UKCC, 1998) and Clinical Negligence Scheme for Trusts (CNST), CTGs must be stored safely. Intrapartum CTGs should be placed in a brown labelled envelope and filed in case notes.

REFERENCES

Gibb D, Arulkumaran S (1992) **Fetal Monitoring in Practice** Butterworth Heinemann Ltd: London

Ingemarrson I, Ingemairson E, Spencer J (1993) **Fetal Heart Rate Monitoring** Oxford Medical Publications: Oxford

Medical Devices Agency (MDA) (1998) **Cardiotocograph (CTG) monitoring of fetus during labour.** Safety notice MDA SN 9813 March 1998 MDA: London

Nottingham City Hospital (NHS Trust) (1999) **Guidelines Policy.** Nottingham City Hospital (NHS Trust): Nottingham

United Kingdom Central Council for Nurses, Midwives and Health Visitors (UKCC) (1998) **Midwives rules and code of conduct.** UKCC: London

INTRAPARTUM FETAL MONITORING ACTIVE SECOND STAGE
Nottingham City Hospital (NHS Trust) Maternity Unit
Review August 1998. Final Version.

- **Prior to commencement of active 2nd stage, 1st stage guidelines apply.**

- There is limited research evidence for cardiotocograph (CTG) standards in the second stage of labour

- Mothers who were monitored intermittently in the 1st stage should have the fetal heart auscultated after each contraction in the active 2nd stage, mothers who were monitored continuously in the 1st stage should be monitored continuously in the 2nd stage. If unable to obtain good quality CTG, record the reason and use alternative method of monitoring. Mothers who have trial of instrumental delivery in theatre should be continuously monitored as soon as possible.

- Mothers who develop meconium-stained liquor, or other complication should have continuous electronic fetal monitoring

- Prolonged increase or decrease in baseline rate should be treated with caution.

INTRAPARTUM CTG CLASSIFICATIONS, DEFINITIONS & TYPES OF DECELERATIONS
See First Stage Intrapartum Guidelines

CLASSIFICATION	BASELINE RATE (bpm)	VARIABILITY (bpm)	DECELERATIONS	ACCELERATIONS
NORMAL	110-150 If CTG normal, baseline 100-109 or 151-160 is acceptable	10-25	Early decelerations with rapid recovery	Not enough evidence to comment on their absence in an otherwise normal labour
SUSPICIOUS	161-170 90-99	5-9 or >25 for 10-20 min	Variable decelerations or any deceleration with slow recovery to baseline after contraction has finished lasting > 2 min	N/A
PATHOLOGICAL	>170 <90	< 5 for > 10 min	Late deceleration or bradycardia > 3 min	N/A
PATHOLOGICAL	"Sinusoidal" trace: smooth wave form of 2-5 cycles/min lasting > 20 min	None	N/A	N/A

ASSESSMENT & ACTION

SUSPICIOUS CTGs

- If the CTG is **SUSPICIOUS**, the following possible causes should be considered and appropriate action taken. If the CTG does not return to normal and has **1 SUSPICIOUS** characteristic and delivery is not imminent, inform the Co-ordinator. If CTG continues to be suspicious, inform medical staff and prepare for delivery. If the CTG has **2 or more SUSPICIOUS** characteristics, expedite delivery. Reasons for any deviation from this standard must be clearly documented.

POSSIBLE CAUSE	CONSIDER	ACTION
Inadequate quality of CTG	* Poor contact from external transducer, Fetal Scalp Electrode (FSE) not working or has become detached	* Check position of transducer / FSE * Consider intermittent auscultation or applying FSE
Maternal Posture	* The mother's position	* Ensure mother is not lying flat
	* Is the mother hypotensive?	* Change position, record BP, give IV fluids if appropriate
	* Has the mother just had a vaginal examination (VE)?	* Change position if appropriate
	* Has the mother been vomiting or had a vasovagal episode?	* Change position if appropriate
	* Has the mother just had a top-up?	* Change position, give 500 ml IV fluids if appropriate
Compromised Fetus eg. IUGR, APH Oligohydramnios	* Is there meconium stained liquor or heavy bleeding?	* Refer to experienced SHO or Registrar. Prepare for delivery
Uterine Hyperstimulation Secondary Uterine Inertia	* Is the uterus over contracting? Is there disproportion? * Uterine rupture/scar dehiscence	* Reduce syntocinon. If not on syntocinon, refer to doctor.
Prolonged breath holding whilst pushing/ Hyperventilation		* Encourage non-directional pushing and adequate inhalation and exhalation between pushes. Avoid hyperventilation.
Maternal Tachycardia/ Pyrexia	* Is the mother anxious?	* Reassurance
	* Epidural in situ	* If temperature > 38°c, inform doctor
	* Maternal infection	* If pulse > 120 bpm, inform doctor

PATHOLOGICAL CTGs

- If the CTG becomes **PATHOLOGICAL**, inform Co-ordinator to deploy relevant medical staff immediately. This should be done **prior** to administration of epidural, spinal or initiation of syntocinon. Prepare for delivery. The Co-ordinator may refer directly to the Consultant on call in the event of suspected mismanagement. The "decision to deliver" to delivery time interval should be as short as possible, but ideally within 30 minutes.

DOCUMENTATION AND STORAGE

- All CTGs should be identified by the mother's name, hospital number and date. The CTG monitor's clock should be checked for accuracy at the beginning and periodically throughout the CTG. Events such as VE, use of bedpan, referral to doctor etc. should be noted on CTG with the time. Staff asked to review the CTG must sign the CTG at the time of review.

- All CTGs should be signed by the midwife on completion, action taken and the type and time of delivery noted on the CTG.

- For legal reasons, to fulfil UKCC rule no. 40 and to comply with C.N.S.T. requirements, **CTGs must be stored safely**. Intrapartum CTGs should be placed in a labelled envelope and stapled to the back of the case notes.

REFERENCES

Federation Internationale de Gynaecologie et d'Obstetrique (FIGO) (1987) **Guidelines for the use of fetal monitoring**. International Journal of Gynaecology and Obstetrics 25:159-167

Gibb D., Arulkumaran S. (1992) **Fetal Monitoring in Practice** Butterworth-Heinemann Ltd: London

Ingemarrson I., Ingemarrson E., Spencer J. (1993) **Fetal Heart Monitoring** Oxford Medical Publications; Oxford

GLOSSARY

AETIOLOGY
The science of causes, especially of disease.

ANONYMISATION
The removal of information that would identify babies, family members, professionals and institutions.

ANTEPARTUM STILLBIRTH
Death of a baby before the onset of labour.

BIAS
Any effect at any stage of investigation that tends to cause results to depart systematically from the true values. Examples include observer bias due to differences among observers recording study results; and selection bias where systematic differences occur between selection of cases and controls.

CARDIOTOCOGRAPH (CTG)
The electronic monitoring of the fetal heart rate and of uterine contractions. The fetal heart rate is recorded by means of either an external ultrasonic abdominal transducer or a fetal scalp electrode. Uterine contractions are recorded by means of an abdominal pressure transducer. The recordings are graphically represented on a continuous paper printout (trace).

CASE CONTROL STUDIES
Case control studies compare exposures in people who have a particular disease or outcome with those who do not.

CONFIDENTIALITY
Information given in confidence may be used only for the purposes for which it is given. There are legal and ethical duties to maintain confidentiality in the NHS. The principles on which CESDI data are collected are that the identities of the panels, the professionals involved, and the mothers and families of the babies which died will be anonymous within the enquiry. As a result it is not possible to release panel reports to outside agencies on any identifiable or individualised basis.

CONFIDENTIAL ENQUIRY
Enquiry by peer groups, including experts in the field, into the cause of, and the factors surrounding, a death where strict confidentiality is observed at all stages of the process. It is a form of clinical audit, with an important difference that the feedback or 'closing of the audit loop' is via reports on the general findings, and not direct feedback to those involved with the individual cases subjected to enquiry.

CONFIDENCE INTERVALS (CI)
A range of values about which there is a 95% chance that it includes the true value. For example, if the stillbirth rate is 5.4 per 1000 total births and the 95% confidence intervals are 5.3 to 5.5 per 1000 total births, then there is a 95% chance that the actual stillbirth rate lies between 5.3 and 5.5 per 1000 total births.

CONGENITAL MALFORMATION/ANOMALY
A physical malformation (including biochemical abnormality) which is present at birth.

CONTROL
As used in a case control study or randomised controlled trial, 'control' means person(s) in a comparison group that differ only in their experience of the disease in question. If matched controls are used they are selected so that they are similar to the study group, or cases, in specific characteristics. eg. Age, sex, weight.

CTG - see Cardiotocograph

DENOMINATORS
The population at risk in the calculation of a rate or ratio. Examples relevant to CESDI include number of all live births as denominator for neonatal mortality rate, and birth weight distribution of all live births for birth weight specific mortality calculations.

EARLY NEONATAL DEATH
Death during the first week of life (0-6 completed days inclusive).

ENQUIRY - see Confidential Enquiry

FETAL DEATH (based on WHO recommended definition)
Death prior to complete expulsion or extraction from its mother of a recognisable fetus, irrespective of duration of pregnancy. After separation, the fetus does not show any evidence of life.

GESTATION
The time from conception to birth. The duration of gestation is measured from the first day of the last normal menstrual period.

GESTATIONAL DIABETES
A carbohydrate intolerance of variable severity with onset, or first recognition during pregnancy.

GRO
General Register Office - the official statistics collection body for Northern Ireland.

HOSPITAL EPISODE STATISTICS (HES)
The HES is a national data collection system, introduced in April 1987 to replace the Hospital Inpatient Enquiry. It covers all specialties and is based on

consultant episodes (a period of care under one consultant). The HES for maternity includes a 'tail' with maternity data. For a delivery the episode includes data for each baby as well as the mother. CESDI has not yet made use of HES data in a routine way in its enquiries so far.

INFANT DEATH
Death in the first year following live birth; on or before the 365th day of life (366th in a leap year!).

INFANT MORTALITY RATE - see Mortality Rates.

INTERMITTENT AUSCULTATION
Listening to the fetal heart using a Pinard stethascope.

INTRAPARTUM DEATH
Intrapartum means during labour, between the onset of (effective) contractions and ending with completion of delivery of the baby. If a baby is born without signs of life, but also without maceration (the skin and other changes that occur a varying length of time after death in the womb), there is a strong presumption that death occurred during labour. There are exceptions in both directions which require judgement on the timing of death in relation to the presumed onset of labour.

LATE FETAL LOSS
For CESDI, a late fetal loss is defined as a death occurring between 20 weeks + 0 days and 23 weeks + 6 days. If gestation is not known or not sure, all births of at least 500g are reported, (at least 300g from 1.1.96). Late fetal loss and stillbirth are distinguished by gestational age at the time of delivery which is not necessarily the time of death.

LEGAL ABORTION
Within CESDI, this is the term used exclusively to describe deliberate ending of a pregnancy, under the provisions of the current law (1967/92 Act of Parliament), with the intention that the fetus will not survive.

LIVE BIRTH
Delivery of an infant which, after complete separation from its mother shows any signs of life.

There is no recognised gestation or weight qualifier in UK law on Birth Registration, so that any birth at any gestation or birth weight which fulfils these criteria should be registered as a live birth.

MORTALITY RATES
i)   **Infant mortality rate**
        Deaths under the age of 1 year following live birth, per 1000 live births
ii)   **Perinatal mortality rate**
        The number of stillbirths and early neonatal deaths (those occurring in the first week of life) per 1000 live and stillbirths
iii)   **Neonatal Death rate**
        The number of neonatal deaths (ie occurring within the first 28 days of life) per 1000 live births

iv) **Postneonatal mortality rate**
Number of infants who die between 28 days and less than 1 year per 1000 live births.
v) **Stillbirth rate**
Number of stillbirths per 1000 of total births (live births and stillbirths)
vi) **Late fetal loss rate**
Number of late fetal losses per 1000 of total births (live births and stillbirths)

NEONATAL DEATH
Death before the age of 28 completed days

NOTIFICATION OF BIRTH
By law all births must be notified to the District Medical Officer (now Director of Public Health) in England and Wales and the Chief Administrative Medical Officer in Scotland and Northern Ireland within 36 hours of their occurrence

NON REGISTRABLE DEATH
A fetus delivered before the end of 24 completed weeks of pregnancy without signs of life

ODDS RATIO (OR)
This is a measure of the excess risk or degree of protection given by exposure to a certain factor. An odds ratio of greater than one shows an increased risk and less than one shows a protective effect.

ONS (Formerly OPCS)
Office for Populations Censuses and Surveys - merged with National Statistics Office to become Office for National Statistics on 1 April 1996.

PERINATAL DEATH
Fetal deaths after 24 completed weeks gestation and death before 6 completed days

PERINATAL MORTALITY RATE - see Mortality Rates.

POSTNEONATAL INFANT DEATH
Death between 1 month and 1 year of age. (28 days to 1 year).

POSTNEONATAL MORTALITY RATE - see Mortality Rates.

REGISTRATION OF BIRTH
A statutory requirement for all births in England, Wales & Northern Ireland within 42 days.

REGISTRATION OF DEATH
Time limit for registration in England, Wales & Northern Ireland is 5 days.

SHOULDER DYSTOCIA

Shoulder dystocia is used to describe a range of difficulties encountered in the delivery of the baby's shoulders. Discrepancies in the definition and the use of terms such as 'mild' or 'severe shoulder dystocia' have led to variations in reported incidence.

STILLBIRTH

i)   Legal definition: England and Wales
        A child which has issued forth from its mother after the 24th week of pregnancy and which did not at any time after being completely expelled from its mother breathe or show any other signs of life

ii)   Legal Definition: Northern Ireland
        A stillbirth 'means the complete expulsion from its mother after the 24th week of pregnancy of a child which did not at anytime after being completely expelled or extracted breathe or show any other evidence of life'.

SUDDEN INFANT DEATH SYNDROME (SIDS)

(1969 Seattle definition): The sudden death of an infant or young child, which is unexpected by history, and in which a thorough postmortem examination fails to demonstrate an adequate cause of death.

With few exceptions SIDS occurs in the first year of life. It is also known as cot death.

SUDDEN UNEXPECTED DEATHS IN INFANCY

A sudden death, unexpected from the previous history. The term is applied to other age groups as well as to a small number of deaths in infancy and early childhood. It includes both explained and unexplained.

TRACES - see Cardiotocograph